THE
Hair Braider's
SECRET REFERENCE MANUAL

The
Hair Braider's
SECRET REFERENCE MANUAL

Diana K. Mitchell

iUniverse, Inc.
New York Bloomington

The Hair Braider's Secret Reference Manual

iUniverse books may be ordered through booksellers or by contacting:

iUniverse
1663 Liberty Drive
Bloomington, IN 47403
www.iuniverse.com
1-800-Authors (1-800-288-4677)

ISBN: 978-0-595-52350-4 (pbk)
ISBN: 978-0-595-62404-1 (ebk)

Printed in the United States of America

iUniverse rev. date: 11/19/2008

In the name of Jesus, I give praise to God!
Thank you, Father, for first saving me through your son, Jesus,
the Christ, and for blessing me to complete this work!

For my mother, Geneva: Thank you for sparking the need for
knowledge in me. You are my inspiration!

For my sister, Donna: Thank you for taking the time to review
this work and provide constructive criticism, especially during the
early rewrites. You mean the world to me!

For my niece, Lauryn: Thank you for trusting me with your
hair and for allowing me to test certain concepts in this book,
which work for me, on you. You're the greatest!

Table of Contents

Illustrations

Acknowledgments

I was blessed to have this book reviewed by the following people, and I would like to thank them for their reviews, which are printed on the front and back covers:

Mr. John Paul DeJoria, Chairman and CEO, John Paul Mitchell Systems (Paul Mitchell Salon Hair Care). www.paulmitchell.com

Mr. Curtis Davis, COO, BioCare Labs. www.biocarelabs.com

Dr. Eunice M. Dudley, Dudley Products, Inc., and Dudley Beauty School System. www.dudleyq.com

In addition, I'd like to thank Margie Wagner-Clews of Empire Education Group, and her assistant. I have never conducted an event as large as Empire's annual "National Competition and Hair Show." The largest event that I have ever coordinated consisted of 50 individuals, and I was tired for weeks after that event. I do not want to imagine how exhausted you all must have been after coordinating and hosting an event for over 3,000 professionals. Although timing was not on our side, I do appreciate your allowing me to send you a prepress hardcopy for review. I enjoyed speaking with both of you over the phone, too.

None of you had to accept my phone calls, read my e-mails, or respond to me in any way, so I thank you for reviewing my work, and encouraging me. I would also like to thank your assistants, who were so gracious and kind to me throughout our communications.

I also want to express my gratitude to a friend and prayer warrior, Linda McCall. Thank you for taking time out to review this work and offer me constructive criticism! Your suggestions on how to make the book read better visually have been invaluable. Knowing all that you do for your family, and others, I am even more grateful that you found time to help me with this work.

I am grateful for everyone at iUniverse, too. I want you all to know that I appreciate each of you so much! Your suggestions have made this a better book.

I want to acknowledge and thank my readers, too. Every effort within my means has been made to catch typos, and grammatical errors that may be present in this work. Thank you for forgiving any errors that I may have missed, or created during the editing process. Your patronage is very much appreciated.

Diana K. Mitchell

Read Me

Before you attempt to braid your hair, read this book thoroughly from cover to cover. As a matter of warning, for further advice or assistance, I recommend that you visit a local professional skilled in the art of hair braiding and hair care, your physician, or a dermatologist.

Any decision to put into use any information in this book is up to the individual/reader! The author, owner of the copyright, and publisher disclaim any liability for damage/loss, direct or indirect, as a probable cause or alleged cause of use of any information in this book, article, etc.

The views expressed in this work are solely those of the author and do not necessarily reflect the views of the publisher, and the publisher hereby disclaims any responsibility for them.

The author is not a licensed cosmetologist. This book reflects her experiences learning how to braid and care for her own hair. If this book inspires you to braid someone's hair other than your own or your child's, please remember that in many states you must have a cosmetologist's license if you plan to charge someone for braiding their hair.

No portion of this work may be reproduced/copied by any means without the author's written permission.

Understanding Textual Notations

For your reading convenience, certain conventions have been instituted throughout this book:

Δ	This symbol indicates that the specified information should be noted as it relates to children/people with thin hair. When you see this symbol, remember to use less force on the hair. There are only four sections in the book where you will see this symbol used with a heading. Within these sections, this symbol applies to every paragraph under those headings, including any "Take Note" headings.
NOTE:	This is used within paragraphs to highlight special information for you to note.
Take Note	This term highlights several noteworthy paragraphs of information, which, usually, follow numbered lists.
Some Things to Think About	This heading appears at the end of each chapter with a brief summary of things to note before moving on to the next chapter.
Italicized words	Words that may not be familiar to the reader have been italicized. Such words have been included in the glossary. This does not apply to titles of books, magazines, movies, and words or phrases that have been italicized (obviously) for effect.

How To Read Instructional Information

For the reader's convenience, in "Step Two" there are two types of instructional information: visual illustration groups, and text. The same heading title has been used for both text and illustration groups.

People who prefer visual-based learning will appreciate using the instructional illustrations that appear on the left-hand-side pages of this book.

Illustrations have identifiers a, b, and c. Visual-based learners will use these identifiers to follow hair strands as they move through an illustration group.

For simplicity and ease of reading for text-based learners, corresponding text does not mention the illustration identifiers. Corresponding text appears on the right-hand-side pages of this book.

Numbers in an illustration correspond to the numbered bullets in the text version of the illustration. For example, the "African Braiding" illustration group begins with illustration #4, which corresponds to bullet point 4 (step 4) in the informational text on the opposite page.

People who prefer both, text- and visual-based learning systems, will appreciate having both types of instructional information to learn from; taking in only what they need in order to understand the instructional group as a whole.

Message to My Readers

Thank you for purchasing my book! May it be a blessing to you.

I wrote this book to help people who have hair like mine learn how to work with, and care for, the hair that God gave them, and to encourage people like me who may have felt less than beautiful in the past because they did not know how to care for their type of hair. I want to share with you what I have learned about growing and taking care of my own tightly curled hair.

Whether you are the mother of a little African-American girl or boy, by birth or adoption, or you need help for yourself, it is my prayer that you will find something in this book that will be a help to you for years to come!

In the past my hair has been anywhere from one-sixteenth of an inch long to as long as seventeen inches. It's usually one-sixteenth of an inch long after I cut out a *perm* that has gone bad. My perms usually "go bad" after I try to retouch my own hair. So, from that perspective, I want to encourage you to leave chemical treatments, and maybe even hair *pressing*, to the professionals, but learn to take care of your natural hair yourself.

My hair is thick and *tightly curled*. At seventeen inches long, and wet, it can look like it's only two inches long. If I didn't comb it out and plait it before it dried, it would still look as though it were only two inches long. Please remember that this book reflects how I work with my hair. If your hair cannot be described as I just described my hair, it can still be braided, but use caution and test instructions in this book, particularly instructions that refer to adding *extensions* to the hair, to see if you need to adjust them to work with your hair type.

It is my prayer that you will find the information within the pages of this book a daily help to you in styling and learning to grow your hair.

Once again, thank you for your patronage!

1
Introduction

When I was growing up, my mother told me that you have to train your hair in order for it to grow. In other words, growing our African-American hair is something that we have to learn how to do.

I never really understood what that meant until I decided to have my hair braided with extensions one day. Money was tight back then, but I loved the look so much that I decided to braid my hair every week myself.

I braided my hair every week for one and a half years. Ever since that time, my hair has grown like wildfire.

When I looked around me back then, I could see that there was—and there still is today—a need for information such as is contained within the pages of this book. And so I began to write the book.

I completed this work over fifteen years ago and put it on a shelf.

Even though I could see the need, I didn't feel like it was time to publish my work back then. For example, I was friends with a Latina in Virginia, my home state, who was married to a black man. They had a beautiful child together. I remember one day my friend telling me that she didn't know how to care for her child's hair.

She also told me that not even her mother really knew how to care for her daughter's hair. Although I could see my friend's need, I still did not feel that it was time to publish this work.

Now is the time. And, according to an analysis of U.S. Census Bureau "Table MS-3. Interracial Married Couples: 1980 to 2002," same-race marriages decreased from 1980 to 2002, while interracial marriages increased. I think it most likely that more biracial African-American children are being born to women who need help learning how to care for their children's hair.

Although my book is written with African-Americans in mind, I hope members from every race, male and female, will purchase my book and enjoy reading it, as they learn how to braid and care for their hair and their children's hair.

Why Do We Braid Our Hair?

I learned how to plait hair out of necessity. My mother would always plait our hair each morning before we left for school. I remember one morning insisting on doing it myself. When I finally admitted that I couldn't do it myself, and that I needed help, it was too late because my sister and I had to leave for school, and my mother had to leave for an appointment. I had to settle for a makeshift hairstyle that morning that I somehow threw together. It looked horrible. I think that is when I decided to learn how to plait my own hair.

I can't remember exactly when I learned how to braid hair, but once I learned how to plait my hair, I couldn't stay away from the mirror, and I wanted to learn everything that I could about hair. My mother had purchased us a set of the *World Book Encyclopedia* and I nearly wore the spine print off the *H* volume, because I would read the article on hair over and over again. I also remember learning terms from my mother, and her sisters, such as *overhand plaiting*, *underhand plaiting*, and *cornrows*. However, centuries old, braiding is a unique method of styling the hair that has been passed down from generation to generation. So, my mother and her sisters did not invent these terms or techniques, and neither did I. They learned them from their mother, and other relatives, and passed that knowledge down to me. This is the knowledge that I am passing on to you.

The home stylist who originally braided my hair with extensions used a common over-and-go type of method to add extensions to my hair. Although she did a good job, it was obvious that I was wearing hair extensions and I preferred a more natural look, so I began to experiment. The methods that you will learn in this book to extend your braided styles are the results of my experiments; they are what

I have learned through trial and error and, when my hair was too short to hold extensions, necessity.

I've used the terms braids and cornrows, but which is the correct term to use? There is an historical answer to that question that will not be discussed in this book (see the "Further Reading and Study" section). Depending on what part of the country you originate from, the words "to braid" or "to cornrow" are two terms that refer to one particular hairstyling method. *Braiding* is the term that we will use.

Your Hair Is Your Crown

As I stated earlier, African braiding is a centuries-old unique hairstyling method, which has been passed down from generation to generation by women of African descent—like my mother, who also told me and my sister that "your hair is your crown." She always wore her hair in beautiful styles.

My first exposure to braids as a hairstyle of distinction and cultural pride came with a January 1979 *Ebony* magazine article on Cicely Tyson. I remember seeing her on the cover and thinking that she *was beauty*—like my mother—to be emulated. She made braids look so elegant. I knew Cicely Tyson to be an actress who played roles that uplifted, exemplified the mental strength of, and brought dignity to, African-American women. She did not play stereotypical roles, and I thought that she was just fantastic. I still hold this actress in high regard. When I saw her on the cover of *Ebony* with her hair in braids, I remember thinking that if she could wear her hair like that, then it was okay for me to wear mine in braids too. Today that is an odd thought, but back then the African-American community was (and I think to a large degree still is) in the process of defining itself as a cultural group.

At the time of the January 1979 *Ebony* article, braids as a hairstyle to complement business dress, or as a social hairstyle, were frowned upon. It took someone with self-confidence to wear them in any business or social setting. I am so thankful that Cicely Tyson, a high-profile celebrity, was able to be herself and use her celebrity to help African-Americans feel comfortable styling their God-given hair in ways suited for their unique hair type, and in any business, or social setting.

While researching the January 1979 *Ebony* cover to make sure that I had the correct date, I discovered that Cicely Tyson had also appeared, wearing what looks to me to be nonextended braids, on the cover of the March 15, 1973 issue of Jet magazine.

In addition, I've discovered that the April 1975 cover of *Ebony* is also a cover to note. Campus queens in this issue wear every hairstyle imaginable among African-Americans. Likewise, on the cover, each wears a different hairstyle: big, and small, Afros; pressed hair; and one, Janell Marie Richards, wears her hair in beautiful nonextended braids.

After the January 1979 Tyson article in *Ebony*, I remember seeing an article in *Essence* magazine that inspired me, too. The article—in the May 1980 anniversary issue, titled "Black Girls Can Shake Their Hair Now!"—was a radical, albeit brief, look at the history of the braided hairstyle. A beautiful Julie Woodson wearing her hair braided on that *Essence* cover was as groundbreaking as the *Ebony* cover of Cicely Tyson wearing her hair in braids.

I have also been inspired by gospel singer and radio talk show host Yolanda Adams, who, like Cicely Tyson, has worn her hair in braids with such elegance.

Cicely Tyson showed us a different way to wear, and think about, braids—as an elegant hairstyle to be worn with dignity.

After Tyson's appearance on the *Ebony* cover, I remember seeing actress Bo Derek in braids for a promotion for the October 1979 movie *10*. Her appearance in that movie, wearing braids, popularized the hairstyle to the general public.

Within the past few decades, we have seen the braided hairstyle progress from an artistic, cultural statement to a practical hairstyle for a busy lifestyle. Today, women and men from all walks of life enjoy creative and simplistic braided styles for a variety of reasons: cultural; as a way to grow hair longer; as a resting phase for damaged hair; as a beautification or aesthetic grooming tool like makeup, earrings, or fingernail polish; as a practical answer to aid a demanding schedule; and, obviously, simply because the wearer chooses to style her/his hair in braided styles.

Whatever your reasons are for choosing this method of styling your hair, the best way to learn how to braid is to have the attitude that you are willing to experiment and get to know your hair. As a side note: I have learned that hair growth is a byproduct of hair braiding, but to maintain hair growth, you must be willing to make changes to how you care for your hair, based on how it responds to different hair-care products and styling methods, and you must be willing to maintain split-free ends.

Before you learn to braid hair, you should know how to plait hair. This book has been written from the perspective that the reader knows how to plait the hair, which is the basis of all braided styles. However, for those who do not know how to plait hair, a section on how to plait hair has been included following the sections on African braiding and French braiding. The section on plaiting the hair acts to clarify any remaining questions concerning the difference between African braiding and French braiding.

After having worn my hair braided in one form or another, on and off, all of my life, I have found that there are three very important steps to braiding that you should follow in attempting to obtain, or maintain, a healthy head of hair. These steps are equally important; you should not concentrate more on one step than on the other steps.

Materials You Will Need

Step One:
1. *Fiber*
2. Shampoo, wash-out conditioner, leave-in conditioner
3. Hanger and clothespin
4. Combs (wide-toothed or a seamless plastic pick for combing the hair, fine-toothed for parting the hair while braiding)
5. Hair scissors
6. Mirrors, stationary and handheld (use the handheld one in conjunction with a stationary dresser mirror for a view of the sides and back of your head)
7. Satin-like *scrunchies* to hold the hair out of the way
8. Optional: blow-dryer, hair grease

Step Two:
1. Fiber from "Step One"
2. Fine-toothed comb
3. Mirrors
4. Hair scissors

5. Bobby pins and scrunchies
6. Optional: rubber bands, fresh fiber, rubber bands, a ball-tipped *seam ripper* with a safety cover

Step Three:
1. Hair scarf
2. Shampoo, wash-out conditioner, leave-in conditioner
3. Hair scissors
4. Bobby pins and scrunchies
5. Optional: hair grease, rubber bands, blow-dryer, wide-toothed comb, mirrors, a ball-tipped seam ripper with a safety cover, and a boar-bristle brush

   Δ   Use a soft brush for a child's/thin hair, a hard one for tightly curled hair like mine

Some Things to Think About

In this chapter I have tried to stress my reasons for writing this book, and some of my experiences with the braided hairstyle.

My hair really didn't grow long until I learned how to "train" it to grow. When the women of my mother's day said that you had to train your hair, I think they really meant that you had to train yourself how to comb and care for your hair. If I'm correct about that, then I am a testament that they were right. When I started to braid my hair, there were all sorts of myths floating around that braiding your hair would cause baldness. I wanted to make sure that braiding my hair did not leave me bald, so I took pains to make sure that my hair was in the best shape that it could be in while it was braided. And even though I only occasionally wear my hair in braids these days, it continues to grow like wildfire because of the lessons I learned taking care of it while wearing it braided.

Now, with the "Materials You Will Need" list, you are ready to begin your journey in learning to braid, with "Step One: The Preparation."

2

Step One: The Preparation

Your first question is probably: What on earth am I going to do with that laundry list of ingredients at the end of the "Introduction"? The answer to that question is spread throughout this book, and you most likely will use everything on that list. Next, if you plan to extend your braided style, you're probably wondering where to obtain the false hair that you will need. It may be purchased from wig shops, variety stores, flea markets, or swap meets.

The two types of hair used in extension braiding are synthetic and human hair. In learning to braid, I recommend using the synthetic hair because it is less expensive than human hair. Whichever hair you use (synthetic or human) it is best to ask the salesperson for assistance in matching the color of the false hair to that of your own hair color. You should plan to buy at least four packages of the synthetic hair for braids that are to be at least midway down your back. For longer braids, you should plan to buy twice as much synthetic hair. The first time that you braid your hair with extensions, it's better to have too much and not need it, than to have too little and then have to run out—halfway through the braiding process—to the store to buy more.

From this point forward we will call both synthetic and human hair *fiber*. Also, directions in this book will generally refer to synthetic fiber.

Δ   Another question that you may have before you begin is: Should I use extensions in my hair? I believe that if your hair is thin, or if you are braiding a child's hair, that you should not use extensions. This is because the temptation when braiding thin hair, or a child's hair, is to use more fiber with the hair than necessary, which may cause the natural hair to break off. But continue reading so that you will understand how to use extensions. About one third of the remainder of this chapter deals with fiber; the rest deals with how to prepare your own hair for braiding.

Preparing the Fiber

You will eventually develop your own method for washing fiber. In the meantime, you may want to use the following steps to prepare the fiber for your hair.

1. One or two days before you plan to braid your hair, shampoo and condition *(wash)* the fiber. To do this, remove the fiber from its plastic wrap, but do not remove the bindings. note: If the fiber does not look like a large plait, remove the rubber band binding at the bottom *(free end)* and loosely plait the fiber; replace the rubber band when you finish.
2. Wet the fiber thoroughly, pour a small amount of shampoo along its length, and work up a lather. To do this, hold the fiber at the top *(bound end)* and open and close your free hand along the length of it until you reach the free end. Do this several times, and gently twist and wring the fiber, as you would if you were trying to get a stain out of a blouse or other article of clothing.
3. Once you have worked up a good lather, rinse the fiber using the same method used to work the shampoo through. Follow this method to condition the fiber too.
4. After the final rinse, utilize a hanger and clothespin and hang the fiber indoors to dry. To do this, cut the rubber band binding off the free end only. Unplait the fiber, and hang one of the three strands over the hanger; secure with the clothespin. Do not remove the rubber band binding of the bound end.

Take Note

It is very important that you wash the fiber before using it in your real hair. This cleanses it by removing most dust particles and debris, which can cause itching once the fiber has been braided into the real hair.

If you like, you may use a blow-dryer to shorten the drying time of the fiber. Do not, however, use a comb attachment.

Preparing Your Hair

First, wash your combs and brushes with the same shampoo and leave-in conditioner (or wash-out conditioner) that you will be using on your hair. As with your hair, do not rinse the leave-in conditioner from your comb or brush. Use a towel to remove any excess leave-in conditioner from your comb and brush.

If you are using a blow-dryer to speed the drying time of the fiber, and will be blow-drying your own hair, stop when the fiber is almost completely dry, and wash and dry your own hair. After washing your hair use a towel to blot excess water. Be aware that you will be combing your hair while it is still wet.

Following is how I wash my hair. Until you discover the best way to wash your own hair, you may want to use the following routine.

1. I've found that the best way to wash my hair (natural or *permed*) is to wash it in the shower. If you don't have a shower, try using a shower attachment in the bathtub. The idea is to keep your hair in a vertical position as you wash it, and not bunch it up. If you can keep it in a vertical position, you will have fewer tangles to comb out later.

2. Δ Thoroughly wet your hair and pour a palmful of shampoo into your hands; rub it over your head, patting it into your scalp. Once the shampoo begins to lather in your hair, use a gentle side-to-side scratching motion on your scalp to help remove any *buildup*. Use the gentle scratching motion all over your scalp until it feels clean. Finger-part your hair into halves and wash one half by opening and closing your hands down the length of it; do the other half the same way. NOTE: Pay attention to the color of the shampoo as you work it through your hair. If it isn't white, you probably need to repeat this step after doing step 3.

3. Rinse the shampoo from your hair by gently patting your scalp, and opening and closing your hands down the length of your hair as the water flows through it.

4. If you are using a wash-out conditioner, use the same motions that you used to shampoo your hair—pat your scalp, and open

and close your hands down the length of your hair—to cover your hair with the conditioner and then wash it from your hair.

5. Towel-dry your hair by wrapping a towel around your head and gently pressing it into your scalp; let it sit on your head for a few minutes, so that excess water is absorbed into the towel. Δ A word of caution: Never scrub your head with a towel, because the friction from the scrubbing may break off hairs along your hairline.

6. If you use oil on your scalp, you may want to begin now to *wean* your scalp from its use. Place a small amount of oil/grease/leave-in conditioner in the palm of your hand, about the size of an acorn, for example, if your hair is shoulder length. If you are using a leave-in conditioner, which is better for your hair, you may use more to cover your hair. Gently rub it over approximately one-fourth of your hair, from the ends to just within one-eighth inch of your scalp. Do the rest of your hair.

7. Now begin sectioning your hair with a wide-tooth comb. Make a part down the center of your scalp, from the front to the back of your head. When you run into resistance, remove the comb, and using your fingers, gently separate the hair through the resistance to the ends. Continue to part through to the back.

8. Divide one of the two halves in half, from the top of your head down to your ear. Begin detangling one of these subsections by combing your hair from the ends up to the scalp. When you run into resistance, use your fingers to separate the hairs in the tangle, then continue detangling. Plait this hair and then go on to the next section. For short hair, it may be necessary to divide the subsections into smaller sections. If your hair is three to four inches past your shoulders, it will be easier to comb if you gently pull it out to its length and hold it near the ends in your fist. You will be opening and closing your fist as you comb your hair. Holding longer hair in your fist as you comb your hair will help you to maintain control over your hair, and it may help decrease breakage.

9. The best way to dry your hair is naturally. If you must use a blow-dryer to save time, use it on a low, cool setting. When using a blow-dryer, the less heat the better, particularly if your

ends are damaged, or if your hair is permed. If your blow-dryer has a comb attachment, you may want to begin at the roots, combing through to the ends of your hair. Each time you run into resistance, lift the dryer from your hair and gently comb the remaining hair. It helps to restart slightly, approximately one-eighth inch to one-fourth inch below the resistance. Continue combing until you run into more resistance. This time try restarting midway along the length of hair already blown dry. Replait this hair and go on to the next section.

10. Once all sections are dry, unplait one section and *trim* split ends, if necessary, using a sharp pair of hair scissors. Replait and do the remaining sections.

11. You are now ready to part out the *main sections* of your chosen style. This may be accomplished in one of two ways: (1) Unplait all sections and simply repart according to the main sections of your chosen style; or (2) Unplait the front two sections and repart the hair according to the main sections of your chosen style. Replait this new section, then go on to the next section and do the same, including unplaited hair from the previous section. Continue until all sections have been completed.

Take Note

Never force a comb through your hair. If your hair is dry and badly tangled, try washing it before combing.

Δ   If your hair type is tight curls, never pull it too tightly to the back, for example, and secure it when it is wet with any type of binding (such as a scrunchie), because, as your hair dries, it will most likely tighten over your scalp even more. Over the years, this may cause hair loss. More immediately, it will probably cause a bad headache that may send you running to your physician to make sure that you are not physically ill. Instead, allow any wet hair pulled to the back into a binding to have some slack between the binding and your scalp.

Some Things to Think About

In this chapter I have tried to stress the importance of clean hair and fiber, that you should always gently comb your hair, and that it is very important to start with split-free ends.

With this knowledge, you are off to a good start and are now ready to braid your hair using one of the methods in "Step Two: Methods of Braiding and Extending."

3

Step Two: Methods of Braiding and Extending

At the end of "Step One," you parted your hair according to the main sections of your chosen hairstyle. Now select a section with which to work.

Example: Pretend that your hair has been sectioned, and plaited, in quarters with two sections in the front, and two horizontal divisions in the back of your head. Starting at the back, unplait the bottom section and vertically part it slightly off center. This will be your *main part*. The main part determines the direction the braids are to lay in relation to the wearers' shoulders: horizontal, diagonal, or perpendicular.

Replait one side. Part the loose side again, parallel to the first part. Bobby-pin, use a scrunchie, or plait the rest of the hair to the side out of your way. You now have a thin, or thick if you like, *slice* of hair with which to work.

Take Note

Δ Before you begin braiding your hair, please note that as you complete a braid, you should do a quick check, to see if you have braided your hair too close to your scalp (*too tight*), by smiling and nodding your head up and down and from side to side. If you feel pain doing this, you have braided your hair too tight and should rebraid wherever you feel pain in order to avoid hair loss.

You are now ready to African braid your hair.

African Braiding

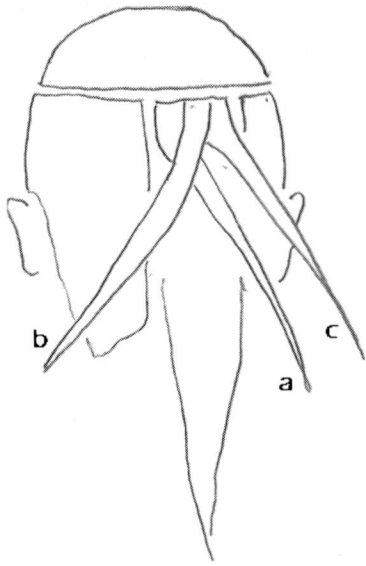

b   c
a

#4

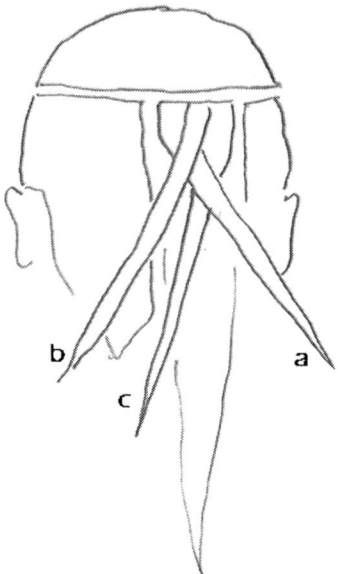

b   a
c

#5

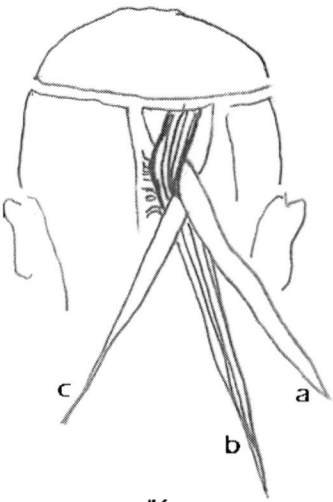

c   a
b

#6

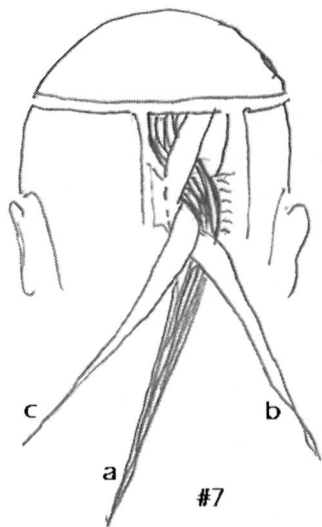

c   b
a   #7

African Braiding

1. Section off a slice of hair to work with, as you did in the introductory paragraphs of this chapter.
2. At the top of the slice, horizontally separate a small amount of the hair (*strip*) from the rest of the slice.
3. Divide this strip into three equal parts (*strands*).
4. Starting with the left strand, **pull it under** the center strand. This strand is now the center strand. What was the center strand is now the left strand.
5. Take the right strand, and pull it **under** the center strand. This strand is now the center strand. What was the center strand is now the right strand.
6. Take the left strand, and pull it **under** the center strand; include hair from the side as you pull this strand under the center strand. If the slice is very narrow, include hair from beneath. This strand is now the center strand. What was the center strand is now the left strand. Note that the hair included from the side or from beneath should be no larger than the strand.
7. Take the right strand, and pull it **under** the center strand; include hair from the side/beneath as you pull this strand under the center strand. This strand is now the center strand. What was the center strand is now the right strand.
8. Repeat steps 6 and 7 to the bottom of the slice, and then simply plait the hair to the ends.

Take Note

When African braiding, what you are doing is plaiting (see the section titled "Underhand Plaiting") the hair down to the scalp by including hair from the side/beneath of a slice as you plait the hair. Practice African braiding until you feel comfortable with this hairstyling method.

Preparing the Cut Bulk

In "Step One," you prepared the fiber for braiding, but there are other steps that you may wish to follow before beginning any of the methods to extend braids. You may find that the following steps expedite the braiding of extensions.

After washing and drying the fiber as described in "Step One," cut one-third of the fiber (*cut bulk*) away from the upper binding. NOTE: If you prefer very long braids, carefully cut and remove the rubber band binding of the bound end and separate one-third of the fiber from the rest of the fiber. We will still call this cut bulk.

Lay the remaining two-thirds over to the side, out of your way.

Δ   Be aware also, and remember, that fiber has weight. A long, thick piece of fiber on a small slice of hair may cause more breakage of the hair than a lesser width of fiber might.

Δ   The cut bulk now may be either divided into widths no wider than one strand of the slice of hair to be braided (for a natural looking braid), or it may be separated as you braid your hair.

If you decide to divide the cut bulk before braiding, simply lay the strands over the arm of a chair or other object to keep them within easy reach while braiding.

Δ Fiber Has Weight

The first time I cut my hair down to the scalp was an accident. After the initial shock, I got used to having very short hair, but after a while, and several intentional scalp cuts later, I decided to regrow my hair. Once it reached a length that was awkward to work with (too short to do anything with, too long to cut again), I decided to extension-plait my hair. I had always wanted to put plaits in my hair that were almost long enough to sit on, and so that's what I did one day.

I left work one Friday with hair about four inches long that looked about one inch long (I was wearing my hair in an Afro), and returned the following Monday with plaits almost long enough to sit on. Most people at work thought that my hair looked nice, and just about everyone asked if it was my real hair. With a wide smile on my face, I told them yes, and that it had grown long overnight. After a few more inquiries, and stares of wonder, I 'fessed up, laughing as I admitted that I was wearing extensions in my hair. What a compliment! I had put the extensions in so well that most people thought that the plaits were my real hair. Even the people who said that they knew it wasn't my real hair kept looking at my hair as if to make sure that they were right.

This was my first time putting such long extensions in my hair. I had previously worn my hair in braids for one and a half years, but had only extended them as far as the middle of my back. I left the long plaits in for about one week. They looked nice, but I didn't want to take the time to rebraid such long plaits.

I just wanted to share that story with you before you proceed to learn how to add extensions to your hair.

Fiber has weight, and too much of it may break your hair off. I was able to plait my hair with such long extensions because I was very familiar with my hair. After years of working with my hair, I knew how much fiber I could add to my hair, and how large I would have to make the parts in my hair in order for it to accommodate the weight of the fiber, without the fiber breaking my hair off.

If this will be your first time working with extensions, follow the instructions above for separating the fiber in preparation for braiding—in widths no wider than one strand of the slice of hair to be braided. As you get to know your hair, and as you practice braiding with fiber, you will learn just how much, or how little, fiber you need to add to your hair, in order for it to appear as if the fiber were part of your hair and not break your hair off.

Extending African Braids

Once again, as you did at the beginning of this chapter, section off a slice of hair to be braided. At the top of the slice, separate the strip from the rest of the hair. You are now ready to extend African braids by one of the following methods that you will learn in this book. I call these methods Under and Around, Under and Go, and As You Go.

Under and Around

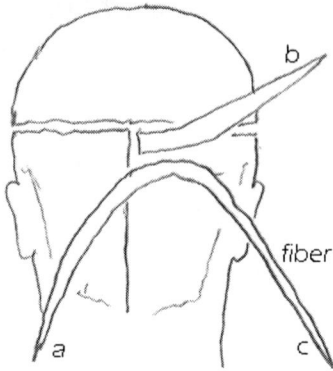

#1

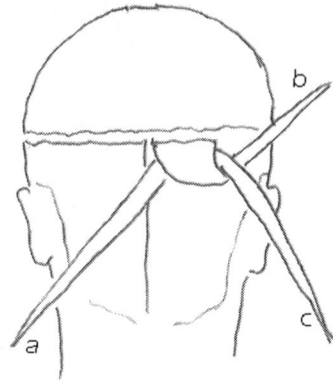

#2

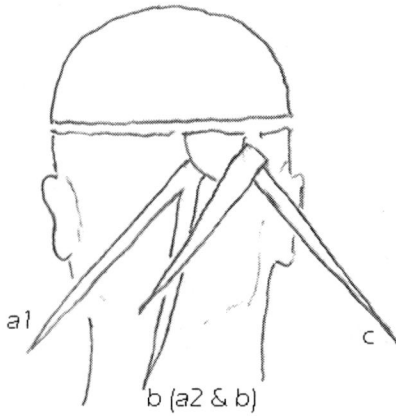

#3

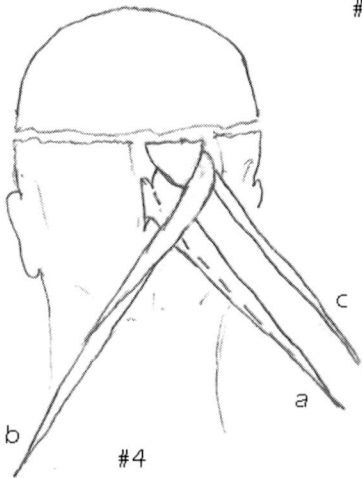

#4

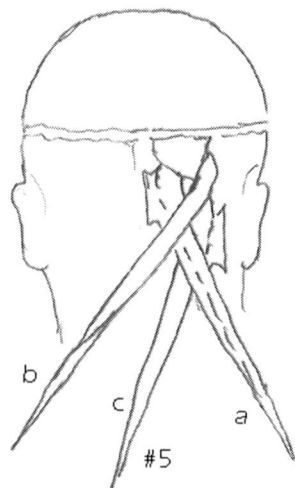

#5

Under and Around

1. Holding the strip at the scalp (*base*) and the fiber at its middle, place the fiber between the strip and the rest of the hair of the slice.
2. Wrap the strip over and around the middle of the fiber. If you are right-handed, the free ends of the strip should be to the right of the base. If you are left-handed, the free ends of the strip should be to the left of the base.
3. If you are right-handed, pull the strip over to the left and combine it with one-half of the fiber on that side. Left to right, you now have three strands: fiber, fiber/hair, fiber. If you are left-handed, pull the strip over to the right and combine it with one-half of the fiber on that side. Left to right, you now have three strands: fiber, hair/fiber, fiber. These strands are uneven. As you braid, even them out by taking a little from too-full strands and giving to strands that are not so full.
4. Starting with the left strand, pull it under the center strand; include hair from the side/beneath as you pull this strand under the center strand. This strand is now the center strand. What was the center strand is now the left strand.
5. Take the right strand, and pull it under the center strand; include hair from the side/beneath as you pull this strand under the center strand. This strand is now the center strand. What was the center strand is now the right strand.
6. Repeat steps 4 and 5 to the bottom of the slice and then simply plait the hair to the ends of the fiber.

Take Note

Δ   When you begin to braid the original center strand, (see step 3) it is a good idea to give the hair part of the fiber/hair (hair/fiber) combination a tug. This will tighten and smooth down the braid, helping to give the illusion that all the hairs (real and fiber) grow from your scalp.

Under and Go

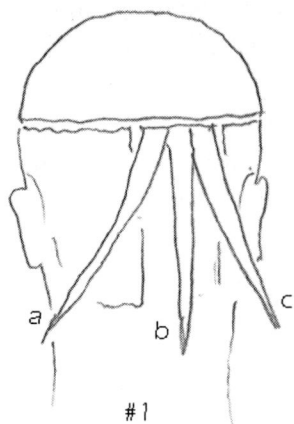

#1

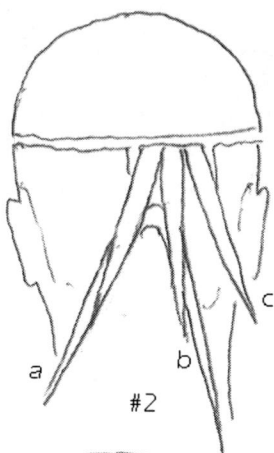

#2

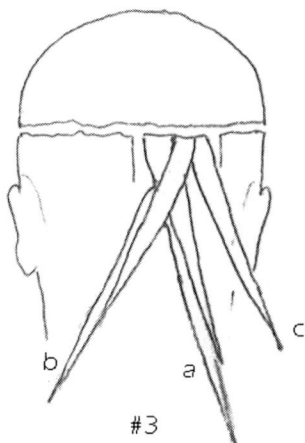

#3

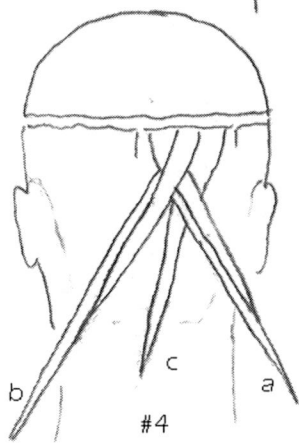

#4

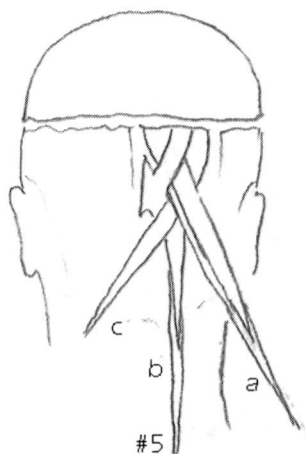

#5

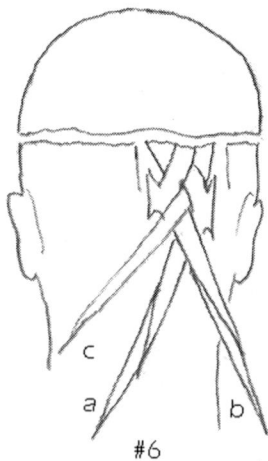

#6

Under and Go

1. Divide the strip into three strands. If you are right-handed, the right strand should be slightly fuller than the other two strands. If you are left-handed, the left strand should be slightly fuller than the other two strands. A variation you may wish to try would be to divide the strip into three equal strands.

2. If you are right-handed, hold the fiber at its middle and place it beneath the left and center strands. You still have three strands: hair/fiber, hair/fiber, hair. If you are left-handed, place the fiber beneath the center and right strands. You still have three strands: hair, fiber/hair, fiber/hair. If you are doing the variation, place the fiber beneath the left and right strands. You still have three strands: hair/fiber, hair, fiber/hair.

3. To do this step correctly, whether you are doing the variation or not, allow the fiber to move as it will, but keep the fiber and hair combinations together. Starting with the left strand, pull it under the center strand. This strand is now the center strand. What was the center strand is now the left strand.

4. Take the right strand, and pull it under the center strand. This strand is now the center strand. What was the center strand is now the right strand.

5. Take the left strand, and pull it under the center strand; include hair from the side/beneath as you pull this strand under the center strand. This strand is now the center strand. What was the center strand is now the left strand.

6. Take the right strand, and pull it under the center strand; include hair from the side/beneath as you pull this strand under the center strand. This strand is now the center strand. What was the center strand is now the right strand.

7. Repeat steps 5 and 6 to the bottom of the slice, and then simply plait the hair to the ends of the fiber.

As You Go

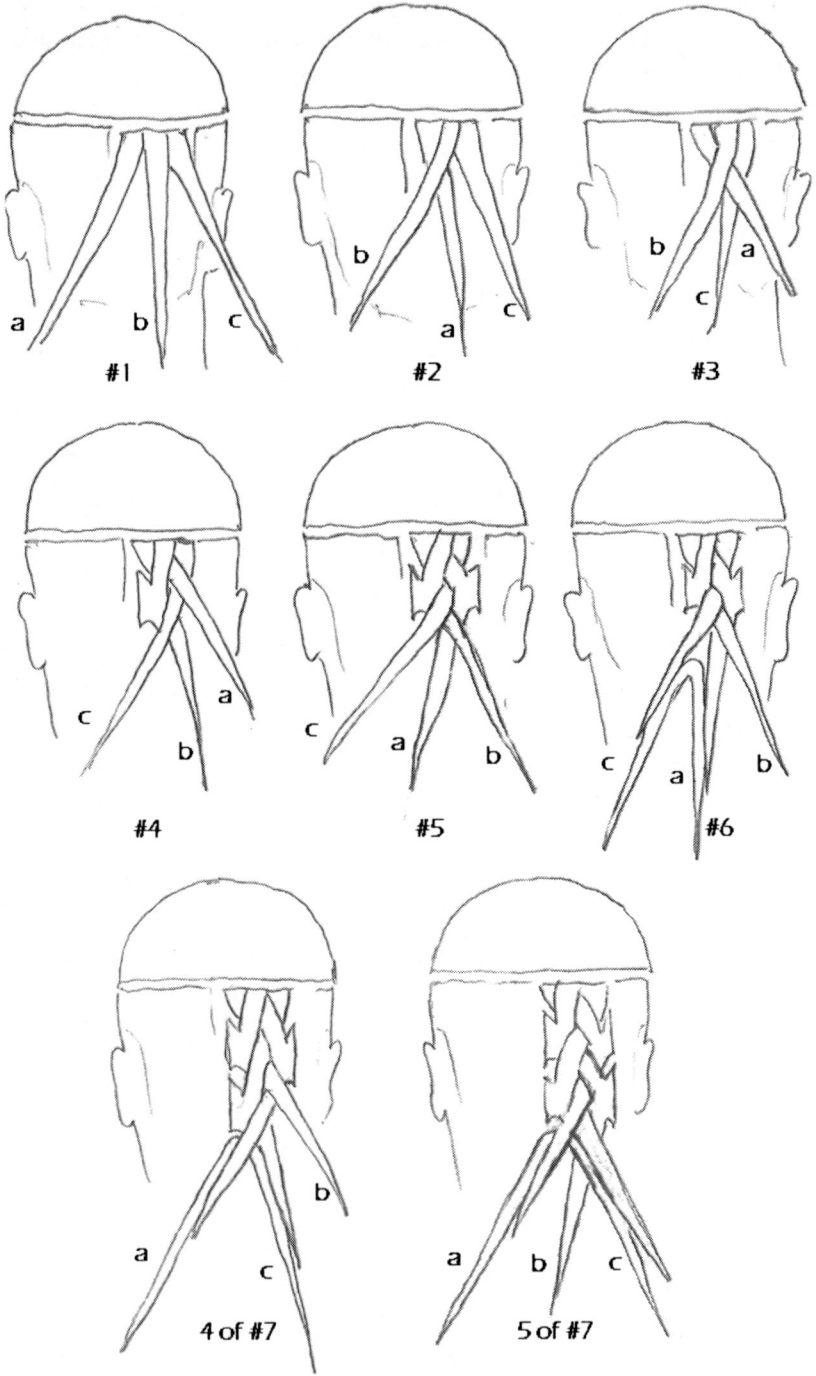

#1

#2

#3

#4

#5

#6

4 of #7

5 of #7

As You Go

1. Divide the strip into three equal strands.
2. Starting with the left strand, pull it under the center strand. This strand is now the center strand. What was the center strand is now the left strand.
3. Take the right strand, and pull it under the center strand. This strand is now the center strand. What was the center strand is now the right strand.
4. Take the left strand, and pull it under the center strand; include hair from the side/beneath as you pull this strand under the center strand. This strand is now the center strand. What was the center strand is now the left strand.
5. Take the right strand, and pull it under the center strand; include hair from the side/beneath as you pull this strand under the center strand. This strand is now the center strand. What was the center strand is now the right strand. Note that steps 4 and 5 are repeated not more than one-fourth of the length of the slice. When this point is reached, go on to step 6.
6. At this point, the extension is added. You should be just about to repeat step 4 (right-handed people), or step 5 (left-handed people). If you are right-handed, take the fiber to be added, and holding it at its middle, place it beneath the center and left strands. You still have three strands: hair/fiber, hair/fiber, hair. If you are left-handed, place the fiber to be added beneath the center and right strands. You still have three strands: hair, fiber/hair, fiber/hair.
7. To do this step correctly, allow the fiber to move as it will. Repeat steps 4 and 5 to the bottom of the slice, and then simply plait the hair to the ends of the fiber.

French Braiding

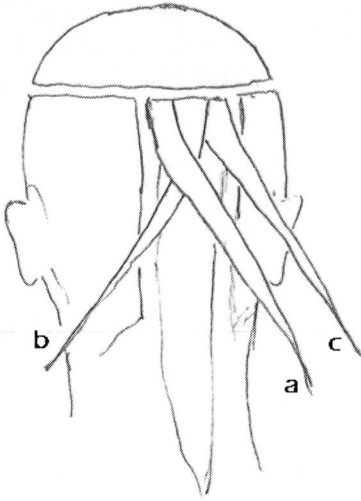

#2

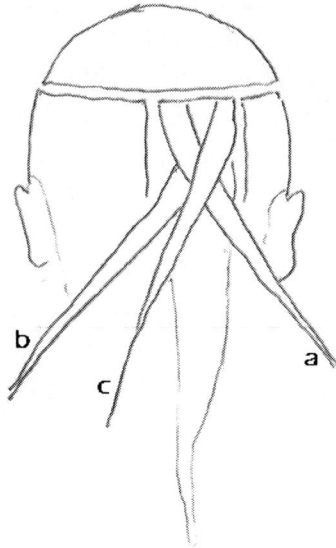

#3

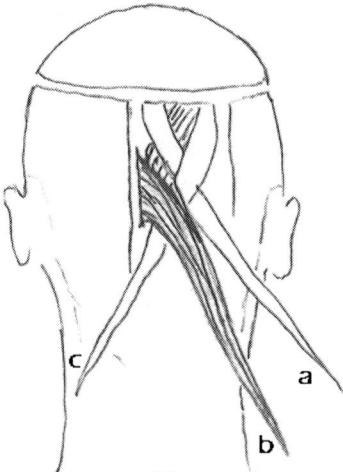

#4

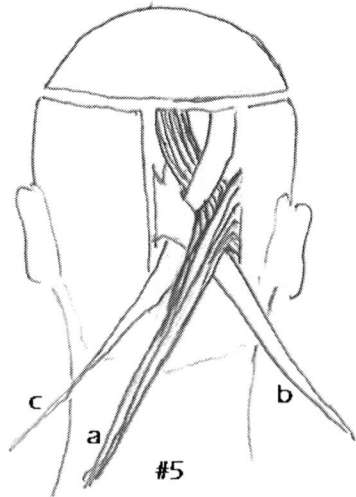

#5

French Braiding

French braids are more aesthetically pleasing when done in large sections.

Example: Part your hair down the middle of your head from the front to the back. Plait one side out of your way. Part the loose section again down the middle of that section from the front to the back. Plait the section nearest to your ear out of your way. Take the loose section, and at your hairline, separate approximately one-half inch to one inch of the hair (strip) from the rest of the slice.

Or, alternatively, to practice the instructions below, you may part your hair as illustrated on the page to the left. You are now ready to French braid your hair.

1. Divide the strip into three equal strands.
2. Starting with the left strand, **pull it over** the center strand. This strand is now the center strand. What was the center strand is now the left strand.
3. Take the right strand, and pull it **over** the center strand. This strand is now the center strand. What was the center strand is now the right strand.
4. Take the left strand, and pull it **over** the center strand; include hair from the side as you pull this strand over the center strand. This strand is now the center strand. What was the center strand is now the left strand.
5. Take the right strand, and pull it **over** the center strand; include hair from the side as you pull this strand over the center strand. This strand is now the center strand. What was the center strand is now the right strand.
6. Repeat steps 4 and 5 to the bottom of the slice, and then simply plait the hair to the ends.

Take Note

When French braiding, what you are doing is plaiting (see the section titled "Overhand Plaiting") the hair down to the scalp and including hair from the sides of a slice as you plait the hair. Practice French braiding until you feel comfortable with this hairstyling method.

African Braiding Versus French Braiding

The difference between African and French braiding is that with French braiding the braid is inverted, because the left and right strands are pulled over the center strand as you include hair from the sides of a slice, as opposed to African braiding, where the left and right strands are pulled under the center strand as you include hair from the side/beneath of a slice.

Extending French Braids

As you did in the first paragraph under the section titled "To French Braid," section off the first slice of hair to be French braided. You also may wish to prepare the cut bulk as described in the section titled "Preparing the Cut Bulk." You are now ready to extend French braids by one of the following methods that you will learn in this book. I call these methods Under and Go, and As You Go.

Under and Go

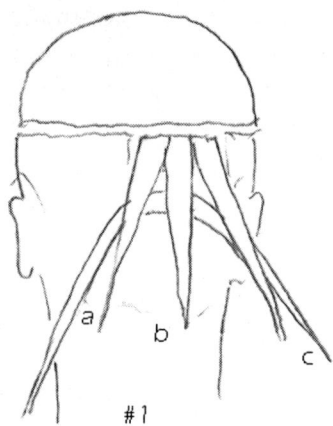

#1

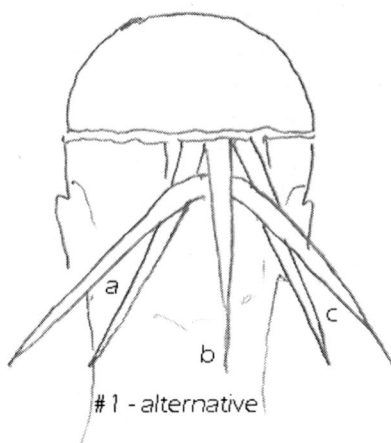

#1 - alternative

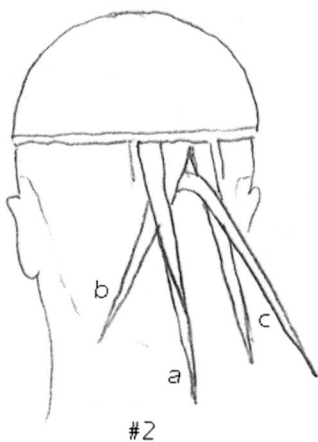

#2

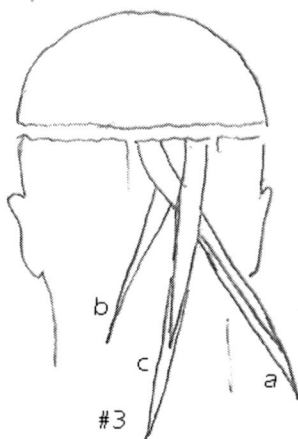

#3

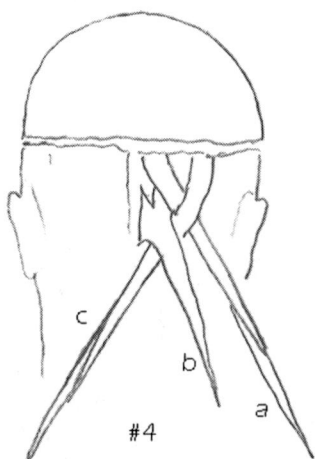

#4

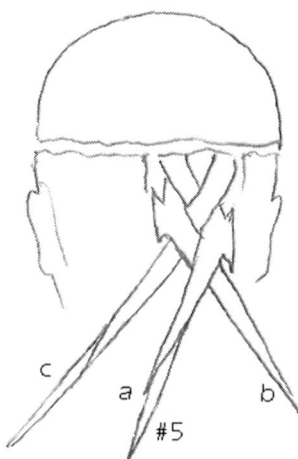

#5

Under and Go

1. Holding the strip at the base, place the fiber between the strip and the rest of the hair of the slice. Combine the fiber with approximately one-fourth of the hair on either side of the strip. Your strands will be as follows: hair/fiber, hair, fiber/hair. Note that, as an alternative, the fiber may lie over the left strand, under the center strand, and over the right strand.

2. Starting with the left strand, pull it over the center strand. This strand is now the center strand. What was the center strand is now the left strand.

3. Take the right strand, and pull it over the center strand. This strand is now the center strand. What was the center strand is now the right strand.

4. Take the left strand, and pull it over the center strand; include hair from the side as you pull this strand over the center strand. This strand is now the center strand. What was the center strand is now the left strand.

5. Take the right strand, and pull it over the center strand; include hair from the side as you pull this strand over the center strand. This strand is now the center strand. What was the center strand is now the right strand.

6. Repeat steps 4 and 5 to the bottom of the slice, and then simply plait the hair to the ends of the fiber.

As You Go

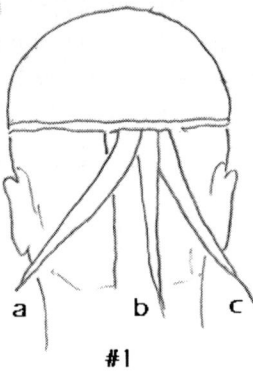

a   b   c

#1

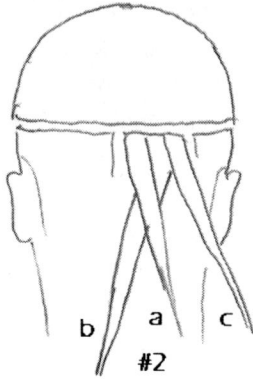

b   a   c

#2

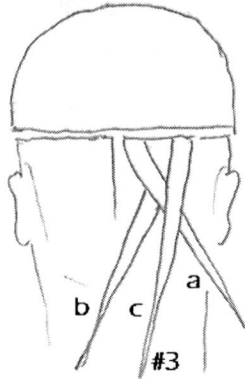

b   c   a

#3

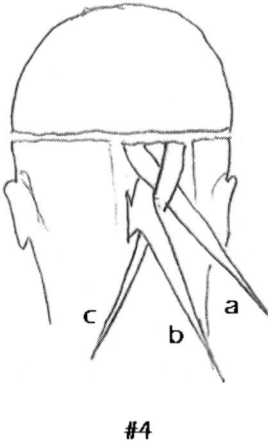

c
b   a

#4

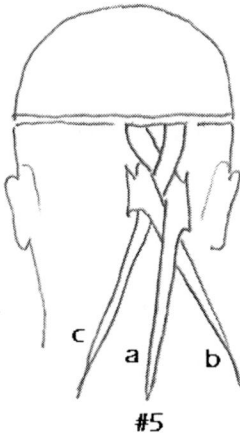

c
a   b

#5

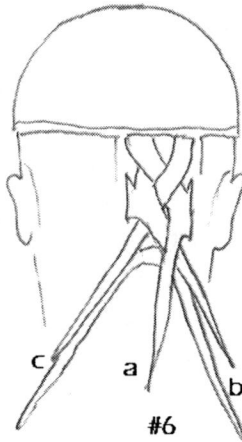

c   a
b

#6

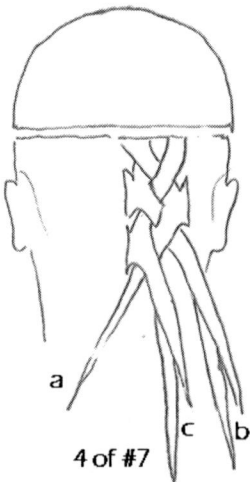

a
c   b

4 of #7

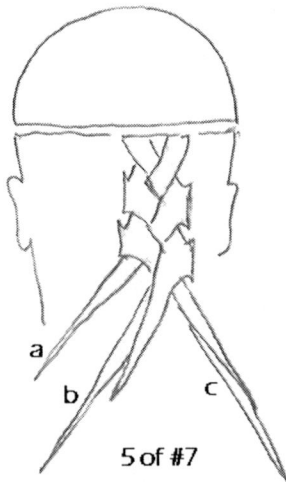

a
b   c

5 of #7

As You Go

1. Divide the strip into three equal strands.
2. Starting with the left strand, pull it over the center strand. This strand is now the center strand. What was the center strand is now the left strand.
3. Take the right strand, and pull it over the center strand. This strand is now the center strand. What was the center strand is now the right strand.
4. Take the left strand, and pull it over the center strand; include hair from the side as you pull this strand over the center strand. This strand is now the center strand. What was the center strand is now the left strand.
5. Take the right strand, and pull it over the center strand; include hair from the side as you pull this strand over the center strand. This strand is now the center strand. What was the center strand is now the right strand. Note that steps 4 and 5 are repeated not more than one-fourth of the length of the slice. When this point is reached, go on to step 6.
6. At this point, the extension is added. Take the fiber to be added, and, holding it at its middle, place it beneath the left and right strands. You still have three strands: hair/fiber, hair, fiber/hair.
7. Repeat steps 4 and 5 to the bottom of the slice, and then simply plait the hair to the ends of the fiber.

Take Note

The process of adding extensions to African braids, or French braids, is difficult at best; however, the more you practice the better you will become.

Plaiting Your Hair

Plaiting is the basis of all braided styles. Let's begin by squaring off a large section of hair to work with at the back of your head. Reach your hands to the back of your head and separate that hair into three even strands. You are now ready to plait your hair by one of the following methods that you will learn in this book. These methods are known as underhand plaiting and overhand plaiting.

Underhand Plaiting

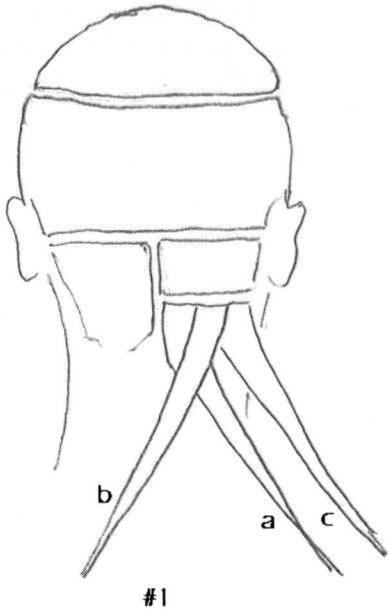

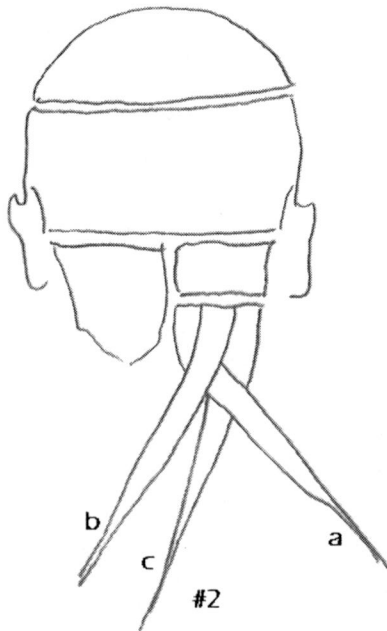

b

a c

#1

b a

c

#2

Underhand Plaiting

1. Starting with the left strand, pull it under the center strand. This strand is now the center strand. What was the center strand is now the left strand.
2. Take the right strand, and pull it under the center strand. This strand is now the center strand. What was the center strand is now the right strand.
3. Repeat steps 1 and 2 to the ends of your hair. NOTE: This method of plaiting the hair is used in all African braided hairstyles.

Overhand Plaiting

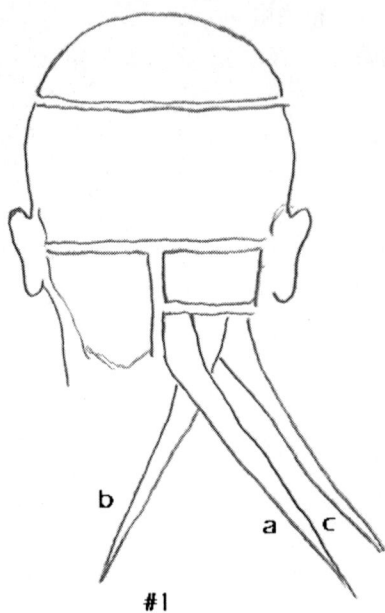

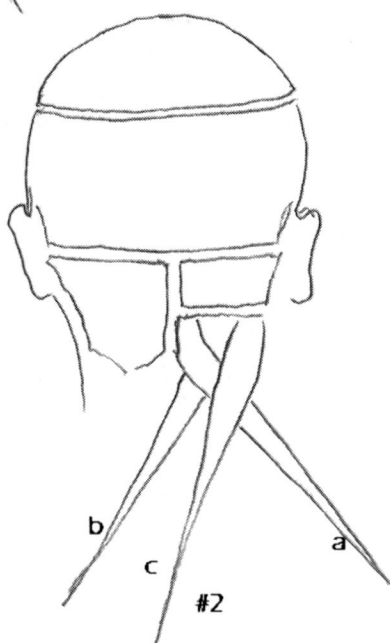

#1

#2

Overhand Plaiting

1. Starting with the left strand, pull it over the center strand. This strand is now the center strand. What was the center strand is now the left strand.
2. Take the right strand, and pull it over the center strand. This strand is now the center strand. What was the center strand is now the right strand.
3. Repeat steps 1 and 2 to the ends of your hair. NOTE: This method of plaiting the hair is used in all French braided hairstyles.

Extending Plaits

You may wish to prepare the cut bulk as described in the section titled "To Extend African Braids." At the back of your head, section off a small square amount of hair (approximately one-half inch is good) with which to work. You are now ready to extension-plait your hair by one of the following methods that you will learn in this book. I call these methods Underplait, Overplait, and Preplait.

I believe that extension-plaiting is an artistic hairstyle, not a wig. I've seen some plaited styles where the plaits have not been plaited to the ends of the fiber, and are so small that it almost looks as though the wearer is actually wearing a wig of loose hair. This can't be good for the hair.

Δ Try to limit the size of your plaits so that you can easily rebraid your hair, and so that the fiber won't break it off during the removal process. I really believe that one-half inch is the smallest amount of hair that you should try to plait, but that is really up to you and what you are trying to accomplish—a temporary hairstyle, or hair growth. Never leave most of the length of your hair extensions (especially the hair/fiber combinations) in an unplaited state. Always plait to the ends of the fiber to avoid hair loss from breakage and split ends.

If you really want to plait your hair in plaits smaller than one-half inch, and leave some of it in an unplaited state, see a licensed professional. Treat this type of hairstyle as a temporary hairstyle for a special occasion. Once the occasion is over, return to that same hairstylist to have the plaits properly removed.

Underplait

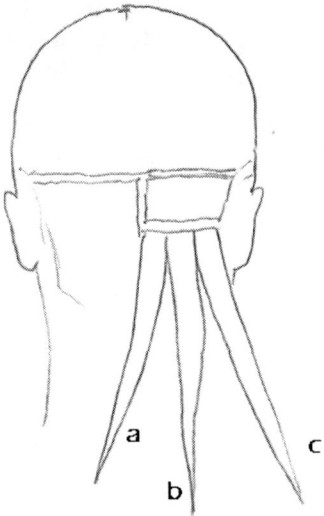

#1

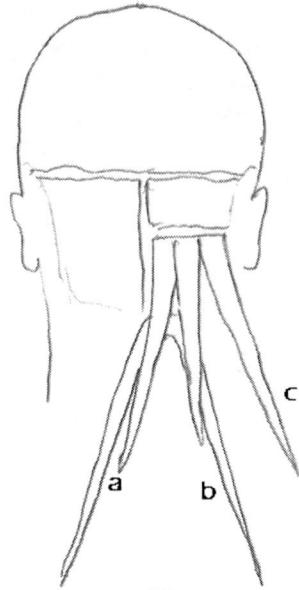

#2

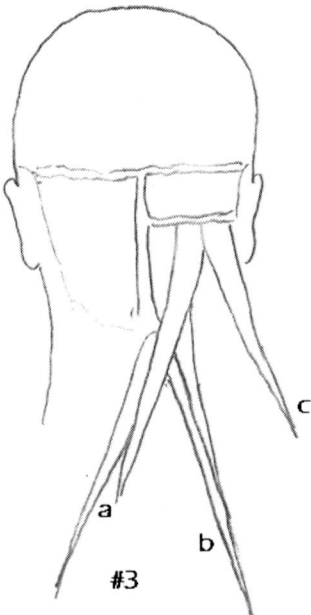

#3

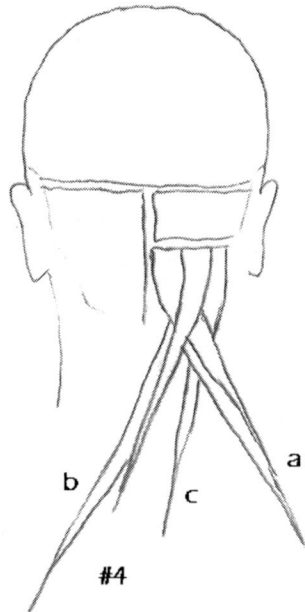

#4

Underplait

1. Divide the section of hair to be extension-plaited into three strands. If you are right-handed, the right strand should be slightly fuller than the other two strands. If you are left-handed, the left strand should be slightly fuller than the other two strands.
2. If you are right-handed, take the fiber to be added, and holding it at its middle, place it beneath the center and left strands. You still have three strands: hair/fiber, hair/fiber, hair. If you are left-handed, place the fiber to be added beneath the center and right strands. You still have three strands: hair, fiber/hair, fiber/hair.
3. Starting with the left strand (allow the fiber to move as it will, but keep the hair and fiber combinations together), pull it under the center strand. This strand is now the center strand. What was the center strand is now the left strand.
4. Take the right strand, and pull it under the center strand. This strand is now the center strand. What was the center strand is now the right strand.
5. Repeat steps 3 and 4 to the ends of the fiber.

Overplait

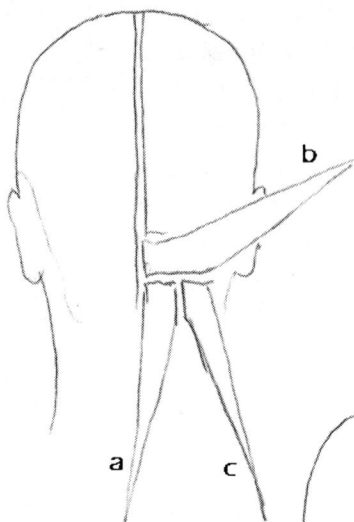

#1

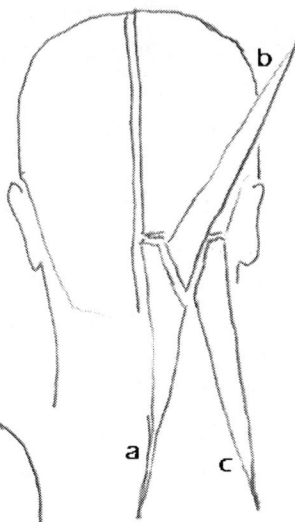

#1 - alternative

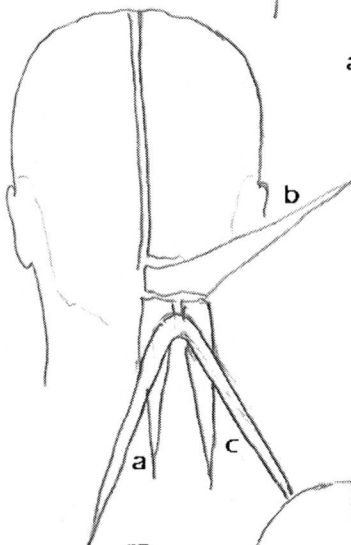

#2

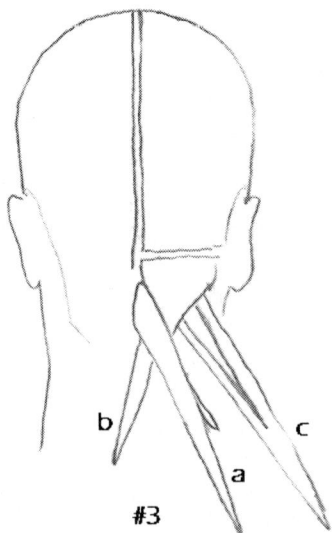

#3

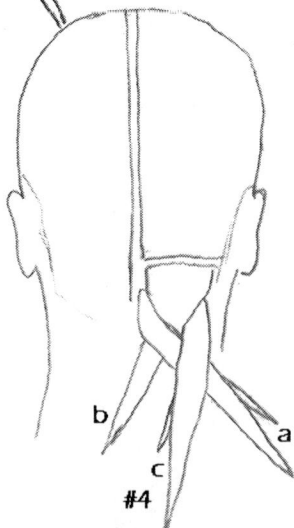

#4

Overplait

1. Using your fingers, horizontally divide the section to be extension-plaited in half. Next, vertically divide the lower section in half. An alternative placement method that you may wish to try would be to diagonally divide the section to be extension-plaited into three triangular sections: part the hair diagonally from the upper corners (start one-fourth the width of the section from the outer edges) down to slightly over the center so that the two diagonals overlap.
2. Take the fiber to be added, and holding it at its middle, place it over the two strands of the lower section you just divided in step 1, above. If you are doing the alternative, place the fiber over the left strand, under the center strand, and over the right strand.
3. Starting with the left strand, pull it over the center strand. This strand is now the center strand. What was the center strand is now the left strand.
4. Take the right strand, and pull it over the center strand. This strand is now the center strand. What was the center strand is now the right strand.
5. Repeat steps 3 and 4 to the ends of the fiber.

Preplait

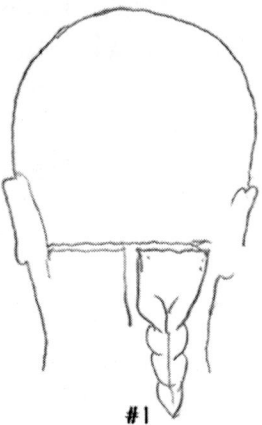

#1

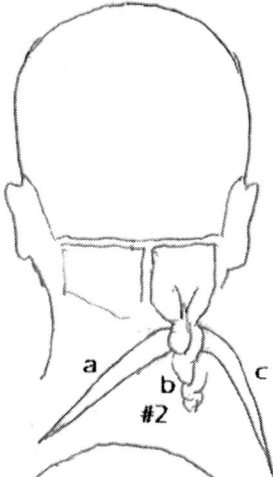

#2

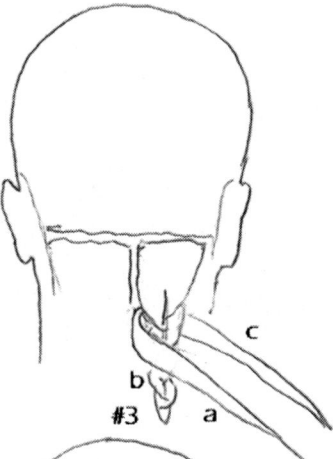

#3

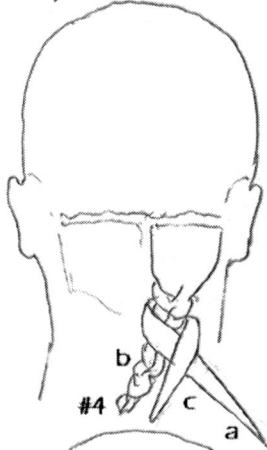

#4

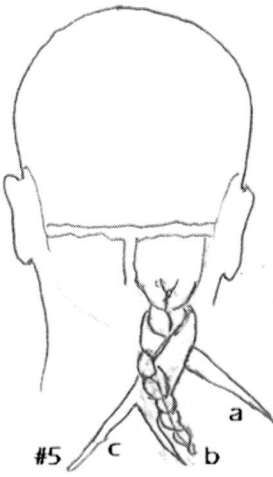

#5

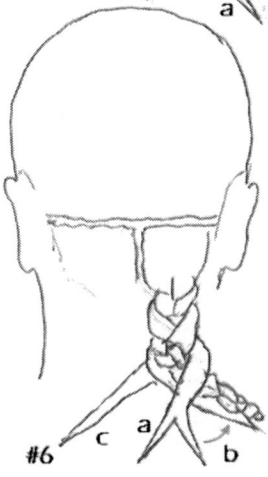

#6

Preplait

1. Plait the section to be extension-plaited using the underhand or overhand method of plaiting the hair. A variation you may wish to try would be to not plait the section to be extended.
2. Take the fiber to be added, and holding it at its middle, place it beneath the hair that you just plaited, at the base. You will have three strands: fiber, the hair you just plaited, and fiber. If you are doing the variation, you will still have three strands: fiber, loose hair, and fiber.
3. Starting with the left strand, pull it over the center strand. This strand is now the center strand. What was the center strand is now the left strand.
4. Take the right strand, and pull it over the center strand. This strand is now the center strand. What was the center strand is now the right strand.
5. At this point, tricky hand motion is necessary. Repeat step 3, BUT, after you have pulled the left strand over the center strand, combine what is now the center strand (the plaited hair) with some of the fiber from what is now the left strand.
6. Again, tricky hand motion is needed for this step. Repeat step 4, BUT, after you have pulled the right strand over the center strand, combine what is now the right strand with some of the fiber from what is now the center strand.
7. Repeat steps 3 and 4 to the ends of the fiber. NOTE: This method of extension-plaiting is the most difficult to do, and the hardest to maintain. It is very useful in extension-plaiting hair that is two inches or less in length. It is extremely important that the wearer whose hair is braided using this extension method does not pull or tug the hair, especially during washing, as the extensions may slip out. Be aware that even if you do not pull or tug your hair during washing, the extensions may still slip out if your hair is very short because the water, shampoo, and conditioner help to loosen the extensions. Steps 5 and 6 are "must-dos" because these steps help "anchor" the fiber to the plait, which helps to keep the extension from slipping out of the plait too soon after the style has been finished.

Take Note

Δ   When using the Preplait method to extend plaits, frequently redoing some of the plaits (more than once week) may be necessary to tighten the plaits in order to avoid extensions slipping out. Also, it is necessary to maintain the real hair by replaiting it at least every two weeks (weekly if you are braiding permed hair) to avoid buildup in the real hair. NOTE: If you do not replait the real hair when redoing the Preplait method, your real hair may *loc*.

Also note that, because the strands start out uneven when you are extending plaits, you must remember to even them out when beginning step 5 in each of the methods of extending plaits.

Some Things to Think About

In this chapter you have learned how to African braid, French braid, plait, and how to extend each of these styling methods. Also in this chapter, it has been stressed that when extending African braids, French braids, or plaits, part of the goal is to do it in such a way that the fiber is not easily detectable.

With any method of braiding or extending, as someone once said, practice makes perfect. Therefore, experiment with these styling methods to find the method that works best for you. For example, if you are right-handed, try the instructions for left-handed people. If you are left-handed, try the instructions for right-handed people to see if you get a better look. The Under and Go method of extending braids under the section titled "To Extend African Braids" offers a variety of possibilities. For example, if you are right-handed, try placing the fiber beneath the center and right strands (as left-handed persons are instructed to do). Note that the left strand would be slightly fuller than the center and right strands. Next, you would start braiding with the left strand as step 3 instructs.

If you are using fiber to extend your braided style, after you have braided all sections the ends may seem uneven. You may want to trim them so that the braids appear neat and somewhat even, but not to the point where they would easily unravel.

Now that you know how to braid, you are ready for "Step Three: Braid Care."

4
Step Three: Braid Care

In "Step Two" you learned to African braid, French braid, plait, and to extend these styling methods with fiber. In "Step Three" you will learn how to care for these styling methods, in particular the care of extensions.

In the "Introduction," I listed some of the reasons women and men of today enjoy wearing creative and simplistic braided styles: cultural; as a way to grow hair longer; as a resting phase for damaged hair; as a beautification or aesthetic grooming tool, like makeup, earrings, or fingernail polish; as a practical answer to aid a demanding schedule; and obviously, simply because the wearer chooses to style her/his hair in braided styles.

I mention this now because you should consider your own reasons for wearing braids/extensions. Your answer(s) will determine how you care for your chosen style. You owe it to yourself to take responsibility for caring for your own hair by noticing how it responds to different hair-care products and styles.

Four factors will be discussed in this book that will affect the growth of your hair while you are wearing braids—with or without extensions. They are: Hair Ornaments and Styling; Daily Care; Weekly Care; and Rebraiding.

Hair Ornaments and Styling

From day to day you may wish to change the appearance of your braids by utilizing the aid of various hair styling ornaments: bobby pins, hair bows, decorative combs, curls, etc.

Δ These styling implements may help to add versatility to what otherwise could be a very monotonous hairstyle; however, they also may cause damage to the hair. To avoid this as much as possible, you should avoid using any ornament that: will snag your hair, is not easily removable for sleep, is painful, is uncomfortable, or puts too much weight on your hair. A good example of the above would be a bobby pin where the rounded tip is coming off or missing.

As mentioned above, sometimes you may wish to curl your braids. When wearing extensions, it is usually best to curl the braids with cold curlers as soon as you have finished a new style or just after rebraiding. If you wish to use hot curlers, it is best if you curl only the part of the braid that is all fiber.

Δ Using Rubber Bands Safely with the CURB System

Ordinarily, I would not endorse using rubber bands on your hair, but my sister has discovered an ingenious, novel, and safe, way to use them on your hair that may help minimize breakage.

If you are in the process of braiding your hair, try to use scrunchies. If you use rubber bands during the braiding process do not wrap them around the hair so tightly that it will be difficult to quickly remove them from your hair.

If you desire to use rubber bands to hold a finished style in place (for example, ponytails that consist of many braids), make sure that you apply your grease/leave-in conditioner to the rubber bands before you use them on your hair, to help minimize breakage.

To remove rubber bands from your hair, or your child's hair, you will need the ball-tipped seam ripper with a safety cover listed in the materials section for "Step Two." My sister loves to use rubber bands on her daughter's hair to hold her loose hairs—and her braids when her hair is braided—neatly together in ponytails. She then wraps stylish bows or ribbons around the rubber bands on her daughter's hair. My niece may lose her hair bows, but at least her hair style remains in place because of the rubber bands.

To safely remove the rubber bands, my sister uses a seam ripper as follows:

1. Hold the ponytail stationary with your hands at the point where the rubber band binding wraps around the hair.
2. Using your fingers, and the seam ripper, gently lift up one of the bands of the rubber band binding.
3. As you use the seam ripper to hold the band up and away from your hair and scalp, gently hold onto the rest of the rubber band binding on the ponytail (so that it does not press into the hair), push the seam ripper up and away from your head, or your child's head. This action will break the rubber band binding.
4. Gently unwrap the rubber band binding from around the ponytail.

Take Note

Using the seam ripper to remover rubber bands from your hair is a great way to avoid hair loss that can be attributed to removing rubber bands from your hair using traditional methods. Breakage occurs when you pull the rubber band into the hair as you remove one band at a time, causing hairs to break at the point of stress on the hair caused by this action; or when you simply pull the rubber band off the hair in one swift movement, which can cause pain, and usually a lot of hair breakage.

You can tell whether or not you have hair breakage from rubber band usage by wrapping one around a ponytail in your usual manner, and then using your hands to smooth the hair lying on your scalp away from the ponytail. If any hairs move away from the ponytail, note the length of the hair from the scalp to the point of the rubber band binding. If the hairs meet up at the point of the rubber band binding, you probably have hair breakage due to rubber band usage/removal, and should start using my sister's system to minimize breakage, and safely use rubber bands on your hair, and/or your child's hair.

For the sake of reference, I'll refer to this system as CURB ("Correctly Using Rubber Bands").

Daily Care

Whenever you have free time during the day you may wish to try a scalp massage. If this is painful, your braids may be too tight. Try rebraiding the area that is painful.

If you wear your hair in braids during the winter months, I recommend that you wear a cap with a satin-like lining, or use a satin-like scarf with a cap, whenever you go outside, or are in a cold area indoors. The cap with help you to avoid a cold and the satin-like scarf will help to keep your braids neat. Also, whenever you sleep, it is a good idea to secure your braids with a satin-like scarf.

Using scarves will help to keep your braids looking neat from day to day, but you must be careful when you remove them from around your head. Whipping a scarf off of your head may "catch" some hairs in the fabric of the scarf, causing split ends to start, or worsen. In order to keep your braids as neat as possible, and avoid split ends, untie a scarf and gently slip it off of your head.

Although hair-care experts usually recommend using silk scarves, I've used cotton ones too. Again, experiment to see if one type of scarf works better for you over another type.

Weekly Care

It is a good idea to wash and rebraid your hair at least once a week while wearing it braided. Weekly washing and rebraiding help to combat the possible buildup of dust, oil, sweat, dead skin cells, lint, and odor. Because these elements can combine to weaken and damage your hair, try not to go more than one week without washing your braids. As a side note, when I am not wearing braids, I usually wash my hair every day during the summer months, and weekly during the winter months. If I wash it daily during the winter months, I make sure to use a scarf and cap when I go outside, or a cap with a satin-like lining.

Eventually you will discover your own method of washing your braids; however, you may wish to use the following method until you do.

1. The best way to wash your hair—whether it is loose or braided—is to wash it in the shower or use a shower attachment in the bathtub. The objective is to not bunch your hair up, but to keep it in a straight-up-and-down position.

2. Begin by thoroughly wetting your hair.
3. Pour your shampoo into the palms of your hands and work up a small lather.
4. Squeeze the shampoo through your braids, gently pressing it into your scalp.
5. Run your fingers up and down the parts, gently scratching in a side-to-side motion, to help remove buildup. As you do this gentle scratching motion, you are gently moving the braids as you scratch so that you also scratch beneath the braids.
6. Separate a group of braids and squeeze the lather down the length of them by intermittently opening and closing your fist down their length to the ends of the braids. Repeat, and then do the remaining sections. NOTE: Look at the color of the shampoo. If it isn't white (or whatever color the manufacturer says that it should be), repeat this step after you do step 7.
7. Rinse the shampoo from your hair using the same motions that you used to shampoo your hair.
8. If you use a wash-out conditioner, condition your hair and rinse the conditioner from your hair using the same motions that you used to shampoo your hair. If possible, it is best to allow your hair to dry naturally.

Δ Rebraiding

After washing and drying your hair, you will notice that your braids seem loose. This is due both to washing and new growth. Rebraiding will help to avoid *matting*, and friction on the new growth from the braids.

You may wish to rebraid the front sections first. The strategy here is that if you cannot complete all sections at one sitting, you can always pull all of the braids to the back of your head into one plait to cover up any unbraided sections, and do any remaining sections later when you have the time to finish rebraiding your hair.

After you have selected the section you would like to work with first, secure all other sections out of your way. When rebraiding, do one braid at a time (the other braids of the section are secured out of your way). NOTE: If you decided to put very long braids in your hair (see "Fiber Has Weight," in "Step Two"), you may want to cut the fiber out of your hair, and use fresh fiber to rebraid your hair. If you can't remember where the hair/fiber combinations begin, carefully unbraid one braid in the back of your head, and when you run into the hair/fiber combination, use it as a guide to cut the rest of the braids to that point.

Until you develop your own method of rebraiding, try using the following method to rebraid your hair one braid at a time.

1. Gently unplait the braid from the ends up to the base. Be especially careful when you reach your real hair. Never harshly pull, tug, or use any type of comb or brush while rebraiding. Patiently and gently work with the braid, using your fingers.

2. If you are reusing the fiber, once you have removed it from the strip, lay it over to the side for now. If you are not reusing the fiber that you just removed from your hair, you should have already prepared the new fiber for your hair according to the "Preparing the Fiber" instructions in "Step One."

3. Gently finger-comb your real hair. When you run into resistance, stop and gently work it out with your fingers. You will see what may appear to be a large amount of hair. This is hair that fell out due to hereditary conditions or your hair's growth cycle, or was broken by you during the braiding/unbraiding process. If you feel that the hair loss is excessive, consult your physician. NOTE: If there is buildup near the scalp, detangle that area first. To do this, for example, if you are detangling plaits, using the fingers of both hands, gently pull the hair (at the point of the buildup) out and away from the buildup. It is usually best to start at the edges of the buildup and work your way toward the middle using a side-to-side motion. Do not use an up/down motion to detangle the buildup. That type of motion may cause clumps of hair to break off. Note that with braids (as opposed to plaits) you may want to try squaring off sections of the slice at a time to detangle, particularly if a lot of buildup is present.

4. If you are using new fiber, skip this step. Finger-comb the fiber so that you can use it again. Holding it firmly and slightly off-center, use your thumb, index, and middle fingers as a comb, running them down the length of the fiber. When you run into resistance, stop and gently work it out with your fingers. When you finish finger-combing this side, do the other side.

5. At this point, if you wish, apply a small dab of grease to the hair of the slice and the fiber. NOTE: Leave-in conditioner is better.
6. You are now ready to rebraid this braid using one of the methods of "Step Two."
7. Repeat steps 1 through 6 for the next braid.

Take Note

Detangling the fiber and your real hair is important, in that it helps to avoid matting.

Δ   Also, take special notice of your hairline. If it, or any other area on your scalp, appears more sparse than usual, you may be braiding your hair too tight, or the fiber may be too thick or long to be supported by the slice of hair into which it has been braided.

After you have rebraided all sections, the ends may seem uneven. You may want to trim them so that the braids appear neat and somewhat even, but not to the point where they would easily unravel.

Δ   If you have been carefully rebraiding your hair for at least three to four months, and you have not noticed any new growth near your scalp, you may want to consult a physician to see if there is any medical reason as to why your hair is not growing. My hair seems to grow anywhere from one-fourth inch to one-half inch a month. It also seems to grow slower during the winter months.

The Final Unbraiding

At one period in my life, I wore my hair braided in the same style, using the same fiber, over and over again, for one and a half years. When the fiber became too short to insert folded even two-thirds its length, rather than in the middle, I decided to unbraid my hair completely.

When taking your braids out completely, unbraid a section at a time, detangling each braid with your fingers. Halfway through the section that you're working on, plait the hairs together, and then continue and do the remaining sections the same way. The object is to have at least four large plaits by the time you finish unbraiding your hair. NOTE: At this point in the process, do not comb or brush your hair.

Δ   Wash your hair with the plaits in and towel dry it. While your hair is still wet, unplait one plait and comb it from the ends up to the scalp. For this, I use a smooth Afro pick with no jagged edges. If you run into resistance, use your fingers to gently work it out. Replait and do the remaining plaits.

If you keep your braids in for any length of time, as I did, be prepared for what will appear to be a lot of hair in your comb. You are using a comb now, and you are combing more than one braid at a time.

Also, your scalp may feel painful for a few days, largely because your hair has been growing in a confined state. And, depending on your hair type and the width of your braids, your hair will seem more textured than usual.

To help your hair readjust to its loose-growing state, try wearing it in large French braids, or large plaits, for a week or more. During this time you may find it easier to wash your hair with the French braids or plaits in while you readjust to styling "loose" hair.

Δ Brushing Your Hair Again

Until your scalp feels "normal" again, it would probably be a good idea to not brush your hair. But when you feel it is okay to start brushing your hair again, keep in mind the texture of your hair, and the strength of your hand.

I have hair that is very tightly curled, so I use a hard boar-bristle brush that is reinforced with nylon bristles. After combing the tangles out of my hair and applying a leave-in conditioner, I'll brush it with my brush—just enough to smooth it out—and then I'll usually either plait it in one large plait at the back of my head, or secure it in the back with a scrunchie.

Also, if you are just getting to know your hair, keep an eye on how you brush your hair. Brushing too hard may break your hair off. Experiment with care to find the "brushing balance" that works best for you. I would recommend that you stay away from the mythical figure of "200 brush strokes" a day. For tightly curled hair (or even permed hair) that can be a disaster.

Hairstylists

Hair like mine can be a handful to take care of when it is in its natural state, so after you have removed your braids for the final time and have allowed your hair to continue to grow in a loose state for some time, you may want to get it permanently straightened. When this time comes, you probably will be tempted to run, not walk, to your nearest hairstylist. Do your homework ahead of time. While you are still wearing your hair in braids, take note of other women's hair and ask them questions about where they get their hair done. If you like their answers, visit their salon, and make an appointment with the stylist in question.

Δ   You will want to allow the stylist to work with your natural hair first. After an appointment, it would be a good idea to ask yourself some questions: Did the stylist comb your hair the way you think it should be combed? If not, did you speak up, and, if it was necessary, share with the stylist how you'd like for her/him to comb your hair? Were you comfortable in the stylist's shop? Did you enjoy working with the stylist? Did you feel as though you could communicate freely with the stylist?

I remember that I once went to see a stylist who, for some strange reason, thought that it was okay to comb my hair as though she were attacking something. She used a hacking motion to comb my hair that, after a few minutes, had me wondering if I would have any hair left by the time she finished, so I politely asked for the comb (as respectfully as I could), and proceeded to comb my hair as though it were the most precious thing in the world. When I finished, I handed the comb back to the stylist, and asked her to comb my hair as I had just combed it, which she did. At the time, my hair was long, and I wanted to keep it that way at least a little while longer, so I had to speak up. Upon leaving the shop, I felt like this stylist had respected my concerns, and she did not get offended when I asked her to comb my hair a certain way. That is the type of person I look for to work with my hair. Of course she was the one with the formal training, but it was my head that she was working on.

Ask yourself, and the stylist, as many questions as you can think of before allowing the stylist that you have selected to work with give you a perm.

Some Things to Think About

In this chapter I have tried to stress that, as with any hairstyle, braided hairstyles must be maintained. In realizing this, you are in a better position to avoid the myths that wearing your hair in braids will damage it, or break it off.

A Brief Recap

Things to Remember

1. *Plan your time*. Schedule in on your calendar time to braid/ rebraid your hair. If this is your first time braiding/rebraiding, plan at least eight hours for yourself so that you can take your time and study your own hair. It may not take you the entire eight hours, but even if it does, you are worth it!

2. Δ *Keep your hair clean*. Wash and rebraid it at least once a week. Try not to go longer than two weeks without washing and rebraiding your hair. When not wearing braids, I'll usually wash my natural hair daily during the summer months, and weekly during the winter months. I have been known to wash it daily during the winter months, too, because I've found that combing my hair is easiest after washing it. If my hair is permed, it usually gets washed only once a week (two weeks maximum) by a hairstylist.

3. Δ *Remember that fiber puts weight on your hair*. A thick piece of fiber on a small slice of hair can cause breakage. This is especially important if you decide to use fiber with thin hair or a child's hair. Therefore, if you decide to use fiber, or wear long, thick braids, remember to take special notice of how your hair responds to the weight of the fiber.

4. Δ *Use the CURB system*. Rubber bands can break your hair off if used improperly. Train yourself to use the CURB system in

order to reduce hair loss and breakage that can be attributed to using rubber bands on your hair.

5. *Know what type of false hair you are using.* Try experimenting with using the different types to see which works best for you. When you unpack man-made fiber you will usually find a large plait that is bound at both ends. The top is usually bound with a rubber band and a bobby pin. The free end is usually bound only with a rubber band. When you unpack human fiber, you will find that the hair is loose, being bound only at one end, usually by a gold spiral. I've always used man-made fiber for braiding.

6. *Avoid using grease directly on your scalp.* It can clog the pores. For my thick, tightly curled hair, I've found that creamy-type leave-in conditioners are best to use.

7. *Prepare the fiber for your hair.* Wash fiber before you need to use it in the braiding process.

8. *Prepare your hair for braiding.* Start with clean hair and split-free ends. If your hair is straight, chemically or naturally, try wearing plaits for a few days before you plan to braid it, so that the hair stands away from the scalp, which makes it easier to braid. You might also try plaiting your hair, washing it with the plaits in, and then allowing it to dry with the plaits in to achieve the same effect. Whenever I went from wearing my hair permed to wearing it in braids—that is if I didn't cut the perm out—I would try to let my hair grow out at least one-half inch before I braided it.

Hair Braiding Tips

1. Remember to treat the fiber as if it were your hair. If you condition your hair with any type of conditioner, use that same condition on the fiber, too, and in the same manner.

2. Δ The closer your fingers are to your scalp while you braid your hair, the tighter the braid will be, the easier it is to insert the extension, and, usually, the more convincing it is that the extension is a part of your real hair. Remember to use caution, and as previously stated, never braid your hair so tightly that it is painful to smile and nod your head up and down and from side to side.

3. Braid with your thumb, index, and middle fingers, and try holding the strands in your fists with the remaining fingers (sometimes the middle finger must also be used here) when they are not being braided.

4. To keep braids neat as you braid them, braid sections of hair from left to right if you're right-handed, or from right to left if you're left-handed.

5. When extending any of the styling methods discussed in this book remember to even the strands out after the extension has been added by taking from too-full strands and giving to not-so-full strands.

6. As you braid your hair, separate the strands through to the ends to keep them from bunching together.

7. Δ For greater control while braiding, I have found it a great help to hold the strands down to the braid/French braid with the left hand and separate the strands through to the ends with the right hand when going, for example, from step 2 to step 3 of the "As You Go" method of extending French braids.

8. Although learning how to braid your hair may seem easy, learning how to move your fingers and use difficult hand motions as you braid your hair may make learning to braid seem twice as hard as it really is to learn. Because I am right-handed, this book has been written from that point of view; however, if you are left-handed, try substituting the word "left" when the sentence reads "right." Where this would be too difficult, and because the placement of the braids is important, I have included separate instructions for left-handed people.

9. Another good idea that I got from my sister is to use a cosmetologist's mannequin head to learn how to braid.

The Secret to Growing Longer Hair

On a ride home from college one weekend, a friend told me the secret to growing hair. She said that every time that you wash your hair, it grows.

At one time, I wore my hair in African braids for one and a half years. During that time I went from washing my hair about every two weeks to at least once a week, and while it was in braids, my hair grew from a little less than four inches to a little over twelve inches.

When I took my braids out, I further tested my friend's theory by washing my hair daily, and at least for me, it seems to be true. So, as I've previously stated, experiment with your hair to find out for yourself what works for you, and what doesn't work for you.

I especially encourage you to wash your hair at least weekly while wearing it braided, and trim your split ends at least every few months. I usually trim my ends once in every three to four months. If I'm having difficulty combing my loose hair after washing it, I know that my ends need to be trimmed. Without fail, after I trim my ends, I find it easier to comb my hair the next time I wash it, and I seem to lose fewer hairs.

Δ   When I'm not wearing braids, I'll usually wash my hair daily during the summer months and weekly during the winter months. If I wash my hair daily during the winter months, I'll make sure to cover my head with a satin-like scarf and cap before going outside, or if I have one, I'll use a cap with a satin-like lining. Even if I don't wash my hair daily during the winter months, I wear a cap to protect myself from the cold. Otherwise I'd be a regular at the doctor's office, trying to fight off a cold, or worse, pneumonia.

Another thing that you'll want to do is to keep your comb and brush clean. Wash and condition your comb and brush at least weekly, using the same shampoo and conditioner that you use on your hair. For one final secret to growing your hair longer, review "Brushing Your Hair Again" in "Step Three."

Maintaining a Healthy Head of Hair

Are you ready to learn how to maintain good, healthy hair growth? Here it is: keep your hair clean, exercise as your doctor recommends, keep your hair clean, eat healthy meals, keep your hair clean, comb and brush your hair with care, keep your hair clean, maintain split-free ends, keep your hair clean, regularly clean your comb and brush, and keep your hair clean.

Think of it like this: if you didn't bathe regularly, how long would it be before other people noticed? Keep your hair clean. Unless your doctor says otherwise, wash your hair at least once a week.

How Do I Exercise?

I mentioned exercising as a way to help maintain a healthy head of hair, so I want to encourage you to consult with your doctor and exercise trainer before beginning any exercise routine. As for myself, I find speed walking to be a great way to lose weight or maintain a healthy weight. I usually walk on a treadmill that has built-in bars that I can hold onto when necessary. Also, I'll usually swing my arms as I walk so that I feel like I'm getting a more complete workout.

I noticed a long time ago that some people only exercise what I consider to be the main part of the body, instead of the entire body. So, in addition to (or usually while) speed walking on my treadmill, I also do facial exercises. If I do the facial exercises while walking on the treadmill, I use the built-in bars of the treadmill to keep my balance as I walk. In addition to facial exercises, I also usually do ankle, toe, wrist, finger, neck, eye, and mouth exercises.

Some Things to Think About

As we leave this chapter, please remember that getting to know your hair and body is the best way to grow your hair longer, and maintain a healthy head of hair.

6
Concluding Words

Considering a Career in Cosmetology?

Nothing sells real hair like real hair. If I can see that you can take care of your real hair, then I believe that you may be able to take care of my hair.

If this book has inspired you to take the next step and go to school to obtain a professional cosmetologist's license, then I encourage you to first take the time to get to know your own hair. Once you begin to understand what works, and what doesn't work for you, take the next step and try braiding someone else's hair. Remember that, as a nonprofessional, in many states you cannot charge someone to braid their hair.

Braiding someone else's hair will give you the opportunity to see if you would like to work with hair professionally. If you find yourself tapping someone on the head with your comb to remind them to sit still as you braid their hair, take it as a hint that cosmetology may not be the field for you. And you probably shouldn't try to braid anyone else's hair. Your sisters, brothers, and friends may not tap you back, but "real" people probably will hit you back, and hard.

Let's say that you pass the "braid someone else's hair" test. What do you do next?

I recommend that you ask to shadow your favorite hairstylist for a few hours. That means that you simply tell them that you are thinking about becoming a professional hairstylist and would like to get a better understanding of the field by watching them for a few hours, or their entire work day. Shadowing is a career technique commonly used in the corporate world.

As you shadow them, remember that they are professionals, with obligations to patrons that must come first. This will be a learning experience for you, so be prepared with your questions, but remember to be polite, and respectful of their patrons' privacy.

If, after shadowing someone, you decide that you do indeed want to pursue a career as a professional cosmetologist, the next step would be for you to locate a school to attend. The person that you shadow will probably be able to help you with this quest.

A Bald-headed Woman

I completed this work over fifteen years ago, and could see the need for a book such as this one at that time, but I didn't feel that that time was the time to publish my work. Back then, God gave me the desire to write this book, but not the desire to publish it right away. I think that I now understand why, but to explain that point, I will have to give you a little background, which includes the next section, "The Purpose-driven Life."

When I was living in Virginia, I accidently cut my hair down to the scalp while learning to use clippers.

It was during the hot summer months, so I couldn't hide beneath a scarf or a hat for very long periods of time, especially at work. I think I'd just moved back up to Richmond from my hometown and had been on a new job only a few months. The first day I cut my hair, someone at work thought that I just had my hair pulled back, but when she realized that I had cut my hair, she (though well-meaning) yelled out in surprise that "Diana cut her hair!"

I knew this person to be a considerate individual, so I knew that she wasn't trying to embarrass me but was genuinely surprised. We had actually been classmates in the past while studying art at Virginia Commonwealth University, and we were surprised to find ourselves working for the same employer. I thought that it was funny that she was so surprised, and we had a good laugh; then I proceeded to explain to everyone that I was trying to cut out a perm that had gone bad (I'd been giving myself a perm about every six weeks). To make the cut efficient, I explained, I'd decided to use clippers. After all, how hard could it be to use them on myself? Up until that time, I had never used clippers in my life. I wasn't sure that I really had the guts to cut my hair again, but I had thought to myself, *just make the first cut from down the middle of your head to the front, and then there's no turning back.* I was right.

The real hard part about having very short hair came when I was standing in line at the 7-Eleven around the corner from my home.

An obviously drunk customer—I can't remember if he was in front of me or behind me in the line—who held in his hands a bottle of liquor to purchase, looked straight at me and yelled out, "A bald-headed woman!"

At first I was petrified and didn't know whether I wanted to yell something back at him or hit him in the face.

He was a lot taller than me, but I figured he was drunk and would probably go down quick, and that would give me enough time to get away before he got back up.

But that was not to be. I had recently rededicated my life to Christ, and I was serious about my Christian walk. I had been baptized as a young girl, but since adulthood I had moved away from God, trying every way to "enlightenment" and the "truth" that I could find, before turning back to rediscover Christianity. Now I was putting dead things behind me, and I was serious about getting to know God.

As I stood there mortified, a strange thing happened. It was as if I could hear God saying to me: "Yes you are bald right now, but so are women who don't have a choice, like those trying to recover from cancer." (I know how this sounds, so if you don't have a relationship with God, or haven't recently dedicated your life to follow Jesus, don't try to figure it out right now.)

Back then I was anything but noble, but when I heard those words, I knew that I didn't have to say anything to that man. I felt God put a peace, and a quiet confidence, in me with those words that I couldn't understand, but I gladly accepted his gift.

I shared this experience with some people at work, and they were so caring. It was like God confirming his words through their thoughtfulness.

The Purpose-driven Life

The Purpose Driven® Life: What on Earth am I Here For? is a popular book written by Pastor Rick Warren. I think that the title and subtitle say it all. Who hasn't wondered what their purpose is in life?

When I wrote this book, *The Hair Braider's Secret Reference Manual*, over fifteen years ago, I was in the middle of searching for my purpose. Part of that purpose is to help others, and in publishing this book to help African-Americans feel more comfortable with their hair type, I believe that I have accomplished a portion of my purpose for being. However, because of my relationship with God, now is the time for me to publish this book. Because of that relationship, I have something more to offer you that will benefit you for the rest of your life, instead of just instructions on how to braid your hair.

You probably noticed that I gave thanks to God in the dedication area of this book. That is because He has bought me through so much in my life. Reading the Bible while I was growing up, I decided that I believed in God, but I always hesitated to call myself a Christian because I did not want to be like "those Christians" that I'd seen around through casual acquaintance. Some were hot-tempered (seemingly all of the time); some seemed to lie; they cursed with tongues that they would also speak blessings with; or, they just seemed boring. It's the boring ones that I should have paid attention to—I've since learned that Christians aren't boring.

If you have considered Jesus and Christianity, but didn't want to be like "those Christians," I would like for you to consider three things: (1) Jesus died for you personally; (2) he said to follow him, not every Tom, Dick, Harry, or Jane who calls himself or herself a Christian; and (3) as someone once shared with me, the church is a hospital, and all of the patients in this hospital are at various stages of healing.

If God has touched your heart right now, ask him in. He is the God who knocks. He will never force you to do anything, because he has given you free will. Just ask him to reveal himself to you, to forgive you of your sins, help you to forgive others who may have wronged you in some way, and to come into your heart.

Does accepting God mean that you will never have another problem for the rest of your life, or make another mistake in your life? No, and no. If anything, life may seem to get harder, but don't get discouraged. Now that you know that heaven and hell are real places, you are better prepared to resist the devil and his little demons. They will come after you with everything that they have in order to keep you ignorant, and let you condemn yourself to that horrible place (hell) when you die.

Be encouraged, read the Bible, ask God to reveal his Word to you, and stay in prayer. (Prayer is a powerful weapon.) I recommend what someone recommended to me: Start with what is known as the Gospels—Matthew, Mark, Luke, and John—and then read the book of Acts, and then the rest of the Bible. I like reading the New International Version (NIV) because it's written in plain English.

There is a verse in the Bible that (to paraphrase) says that faith comes by hearing, and by hearing the Word of God—so I'd like to encourage you to start listening to Christian music on your radio, and ask God to lead you to a church where you can continue to grow in his Word.

Some Things to Think About

I hope that the "A Bald-headed Woman" and "The Purpose-driven Life" sections have given you some things to think about. Remember, it's not what's *on* your head (though important in our society, and to us individually) that matters. In the end, when all is said and done, it's what's in your head and heart, and how you choose to share it, that matters. When God is the head of your life, your heart and God-given mind are your greatest sources of beauty and self-esteem.

You now have all of the tools that you will need in order to learn how to braid and grow your hair to longer lengths, but they will only work for you if you take the time to study your own hair. I've said it before in this work, and it bears repeating: You are worth it!

Now you are ready to try hairstyles of your own. To assist you in this, following (with illustrations on how to achieve them) is a "Gallery of Hairstyles: Designs for Work, School, and Play."

Following the "Gallery of Hairstyles" is "Your Personal Hair-care Diary," which is a specially designed area for you to track what works for you, and what doesn't work for you, as you learn how to braid and train your hair to grow.

Thank you again for purchasing my book. I'll say good-bye here, and God bless you.

7

Gallery of Hairstyles: Designs for Work, School, and Play

The "Gallery of Hairstyles" not only gives the reader ideas for hairstyles, it also illustrates how to section and part the hair in order to achieve them. This aids the braider in learning to read hairstyles worn by others, which may not be illustrated in this book, and apply them to her/his own hair.

To help the reader further understand how to read hairstyles, following the introduction to this chapter are illustrations of a slice, strip, strands, and the anatomy of a hairstyle.

Slice, Strip, and Strands

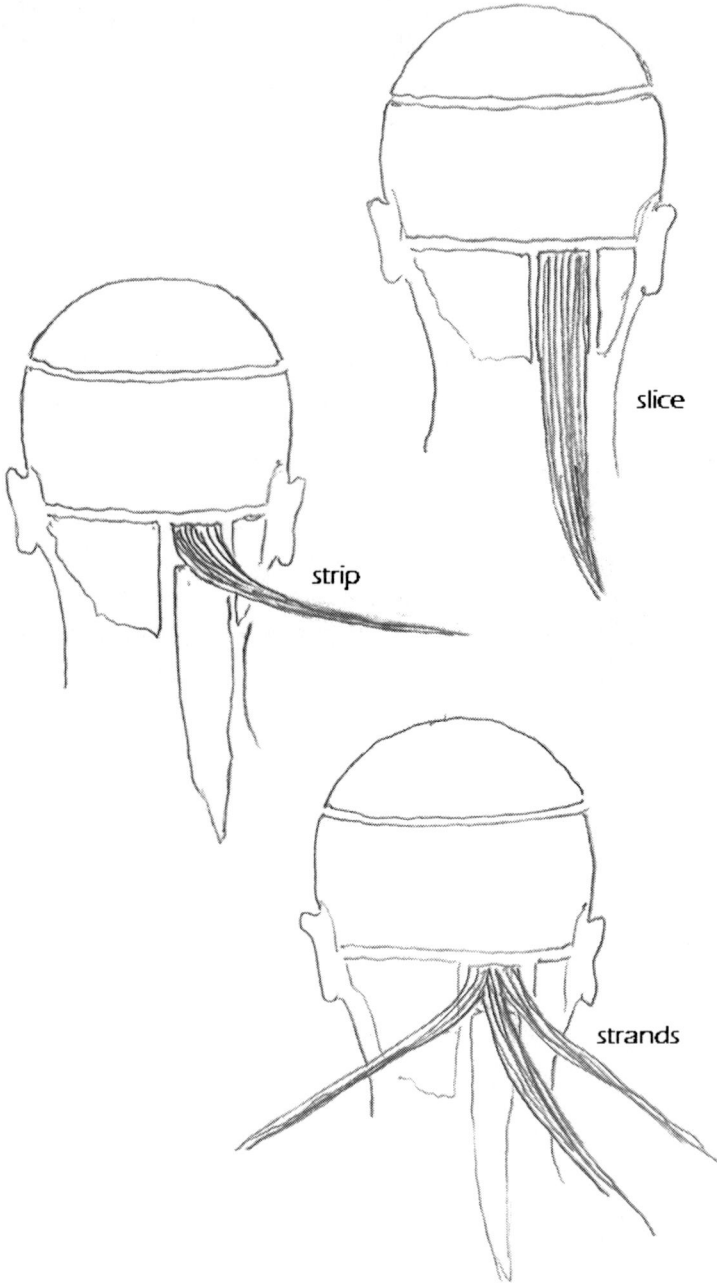

slice

strip

strands

Slice, Strip, and Strands

The slice, strip, and strands are the building blocks of braided hairstyles.

While the slice forms the base—small slices usually being used in African braiding, and larger slices usually being used in French braiding—the strip and strands set the tone of a hairstyle. Short-set braids produce one tone, while long-set braids produce another.

Anatomy of a Hairstyle

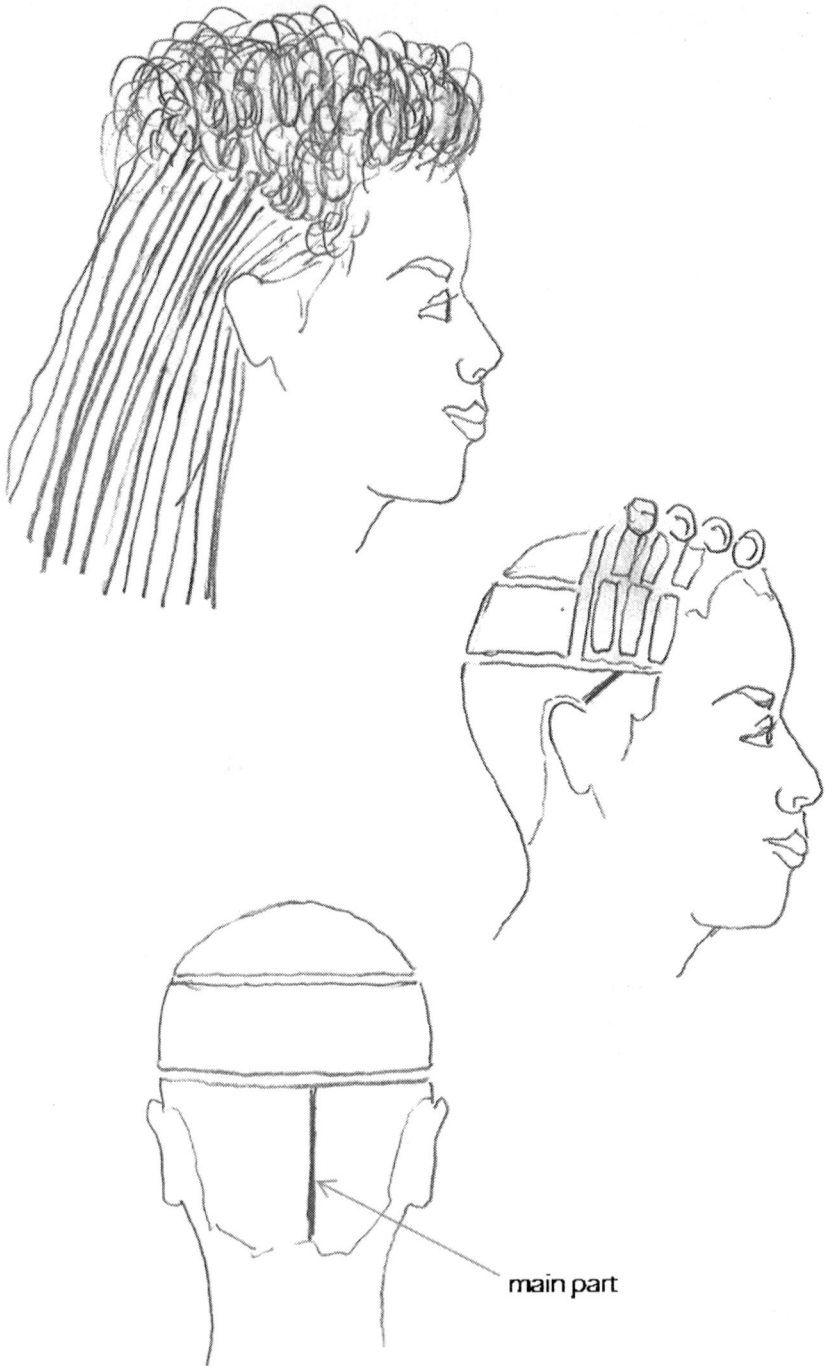

main part

Anatomy of a Hairstyle

For the hairstyle on the left you see:

1. A side view of the finished hairstyle, and side and back views of the blueprint for the hairstyle.
2. The main sections, of which there are four. The front section is curled in the finished style. During the braiding process, this hair is plaited out of the way. It is curled only after all braids have been completed.
3. The main part for the side of the fourth section. It is slanted because all braids on the side are slanted.
4. The main part for the lower back section. Because the entire back is vertical, only one main part needs to be illustrated.

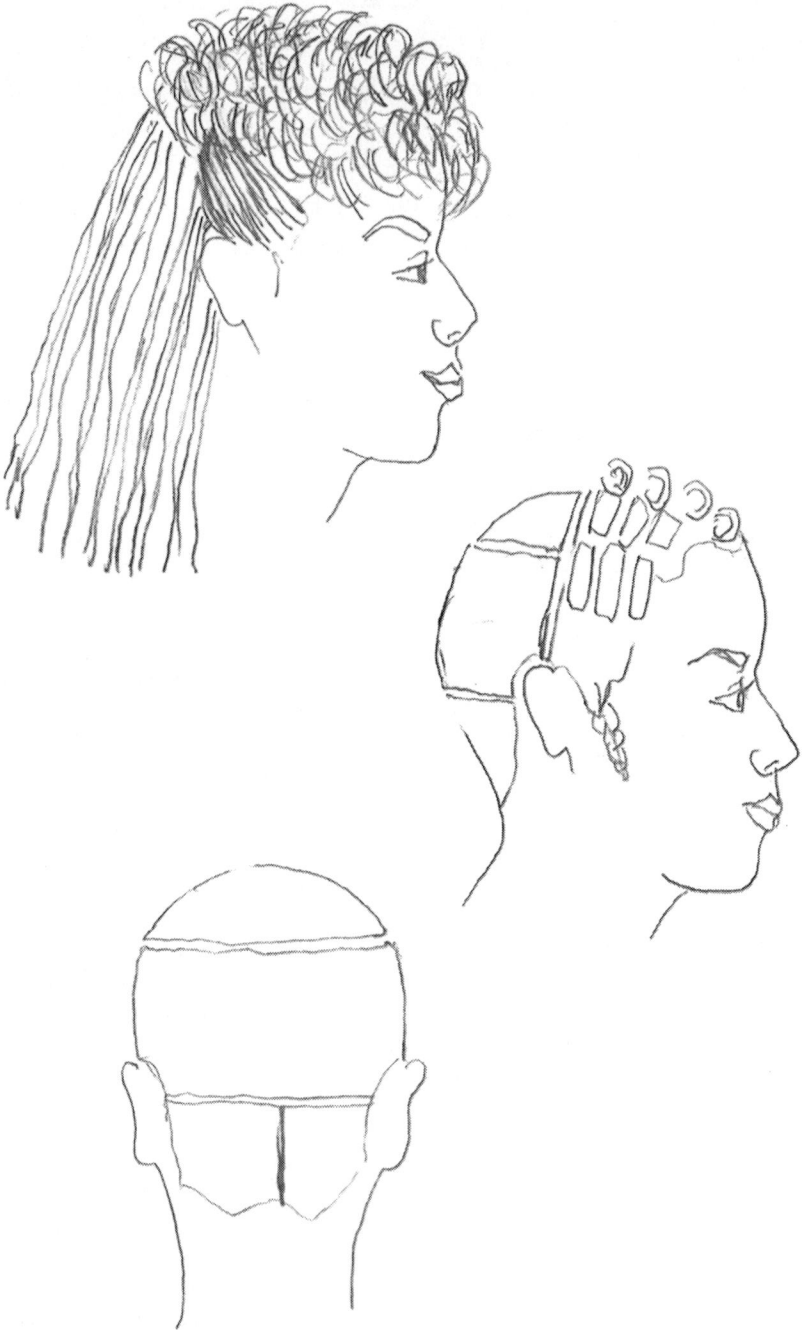

The hairstyle on the left has five sections: two in the front and three in the back. The upper front section is curled in the finished style. The ends of the lower front are curled in the finished style, swept up and bobby-pinned up. All of the front sections are plaited out of the way during the braiding process.

The back sections of this hairstyle may either be in braids or plaits.

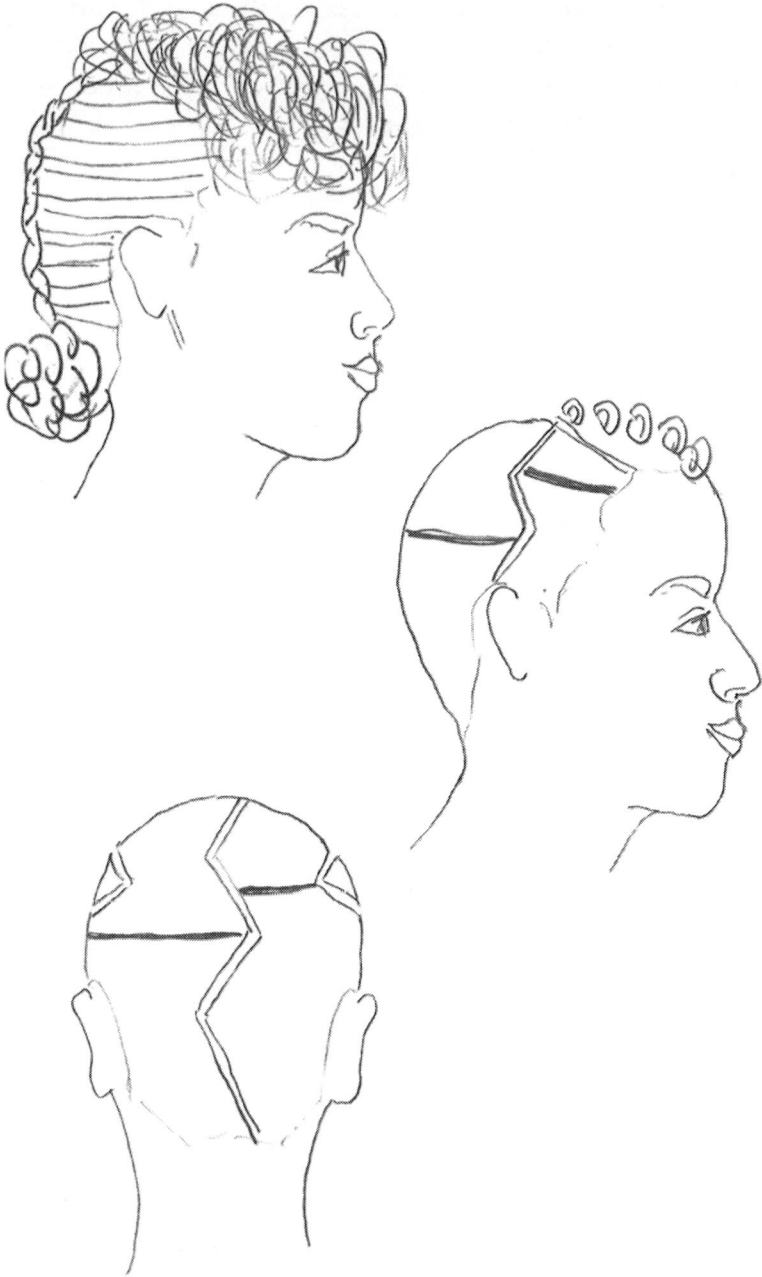

The style to the left has been illustrated as a braided hairstyle with five sections, but this hairstyle would work well as French braids, too. For the French braid alternative, there would be a total of only three sections: the top curled section, and the two French-braided side-to-back sections. Also, remember that each of the French braids would be larger than what has been illustrated for African braids.

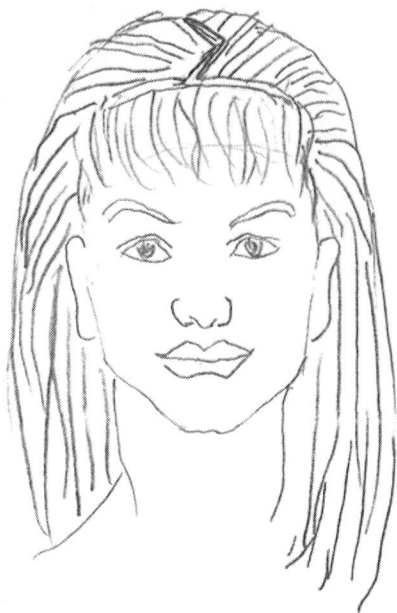

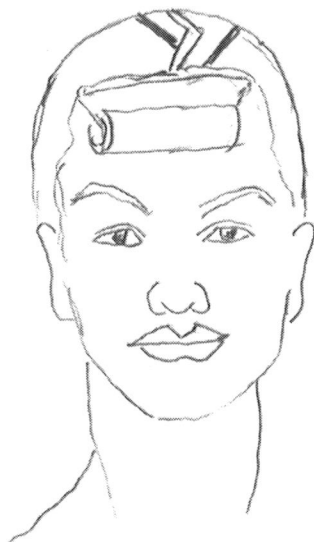

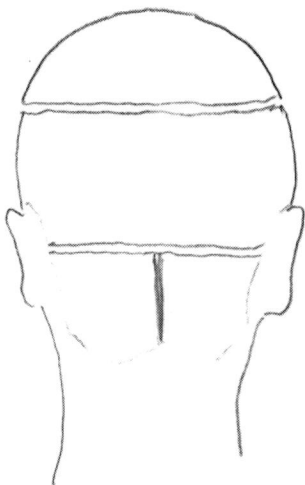

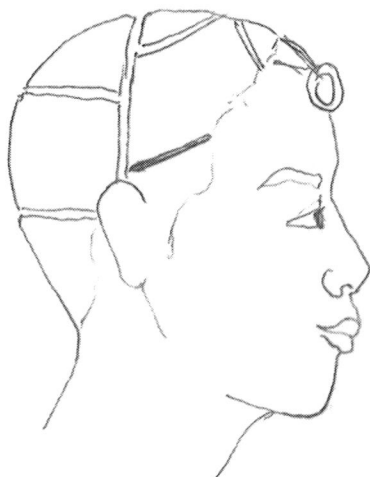

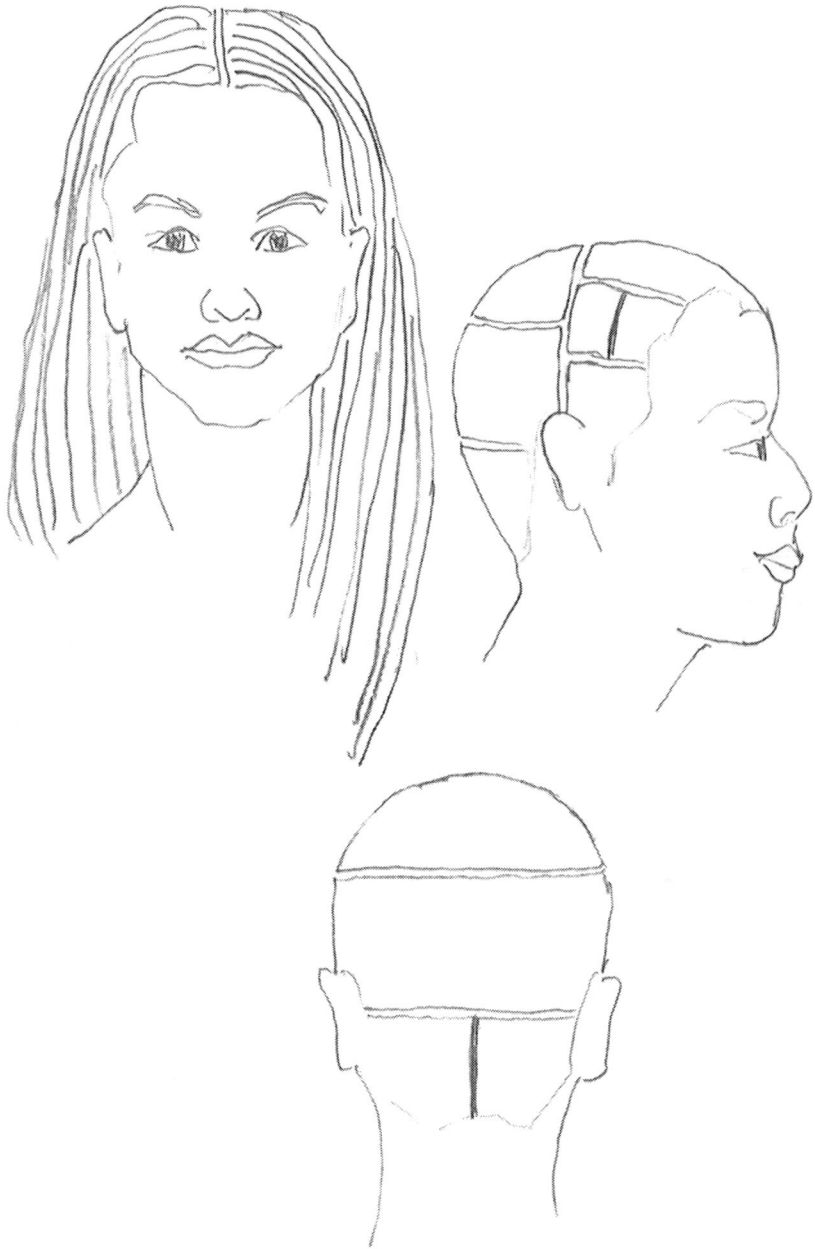

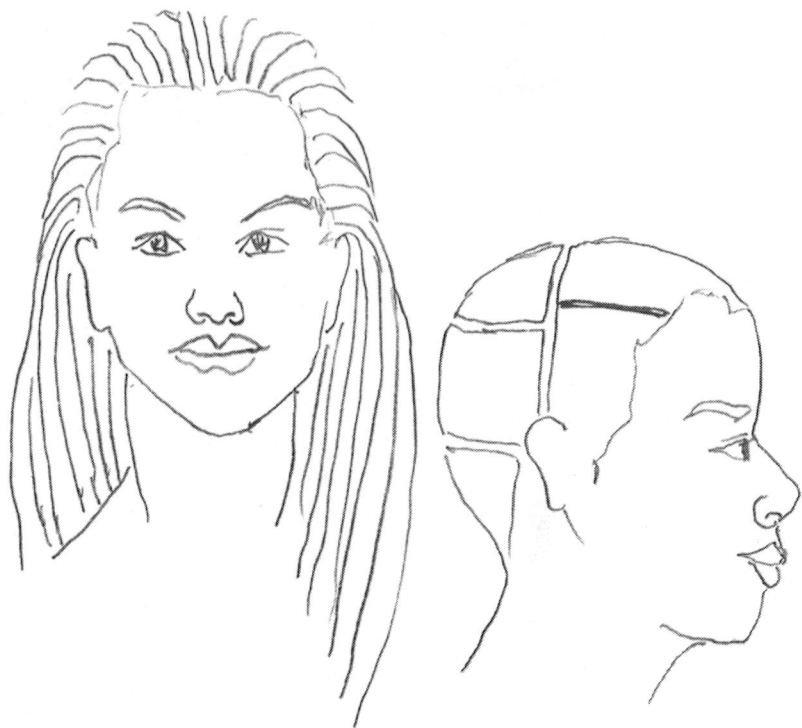

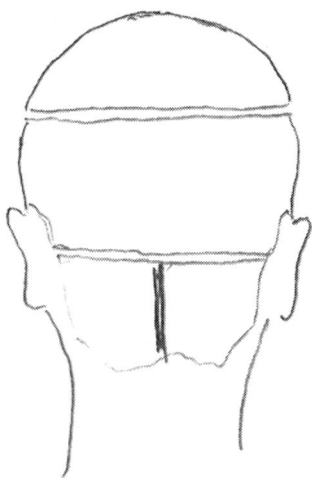

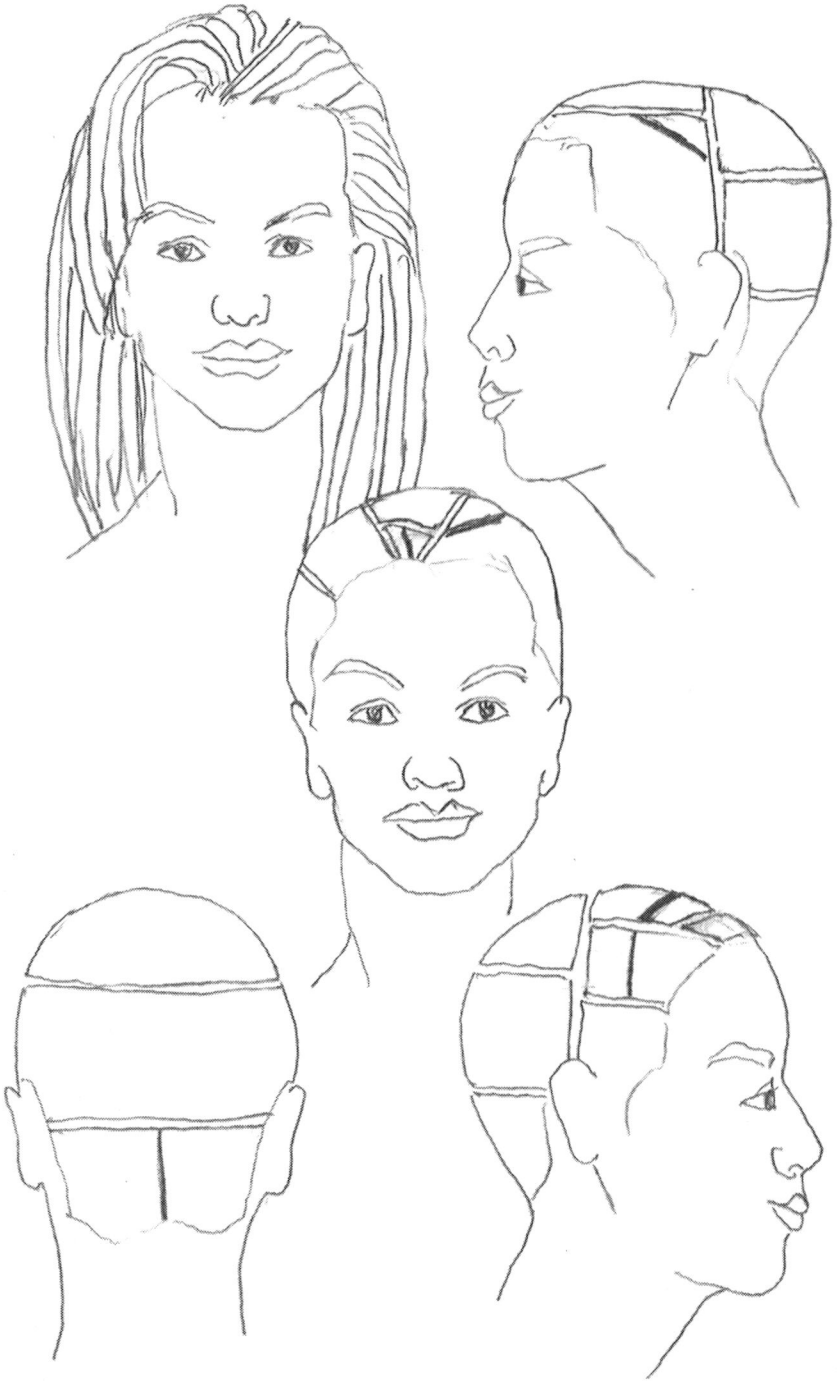

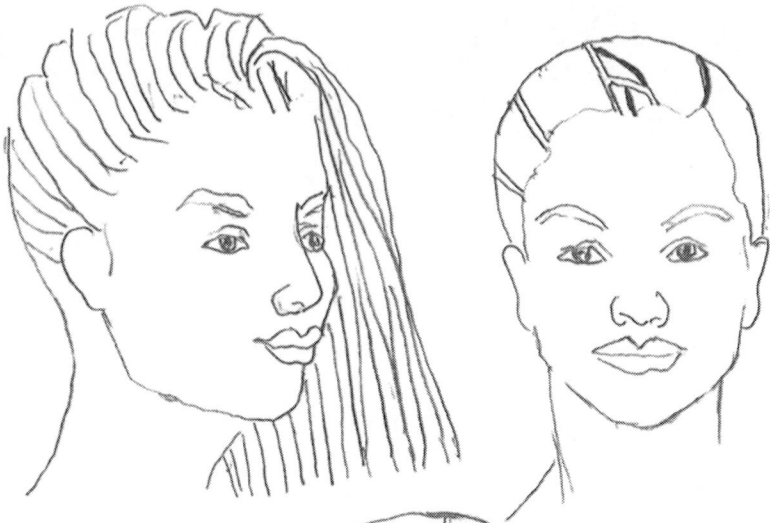

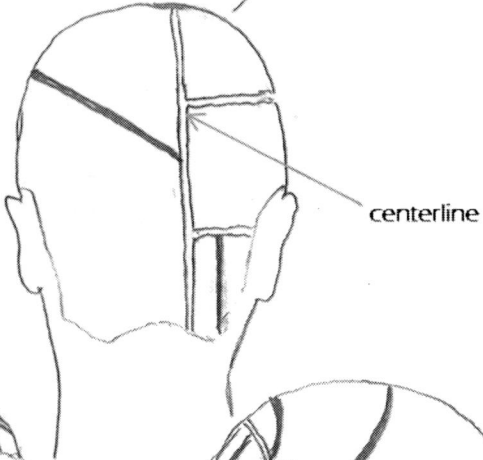

centerline

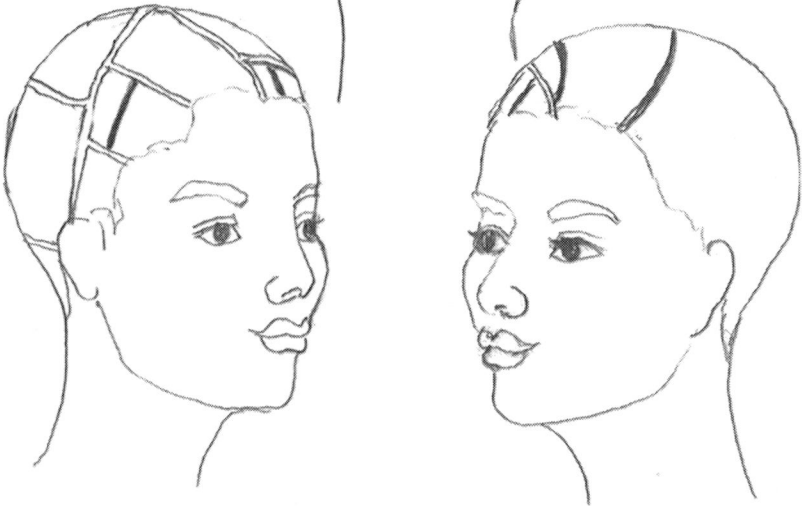

The style to the left has been illustrated as a braided hairstyle with five sections, but this is another hairstyle that would work well as a French braided hairstyle. The hair would be French braided from the left side of the head to the centerline of the back. From that point, depending on your preference, the remaining hair would be in either plaits or braids. Test using braids and plaits to see what look (braids or plaits) you prefer.

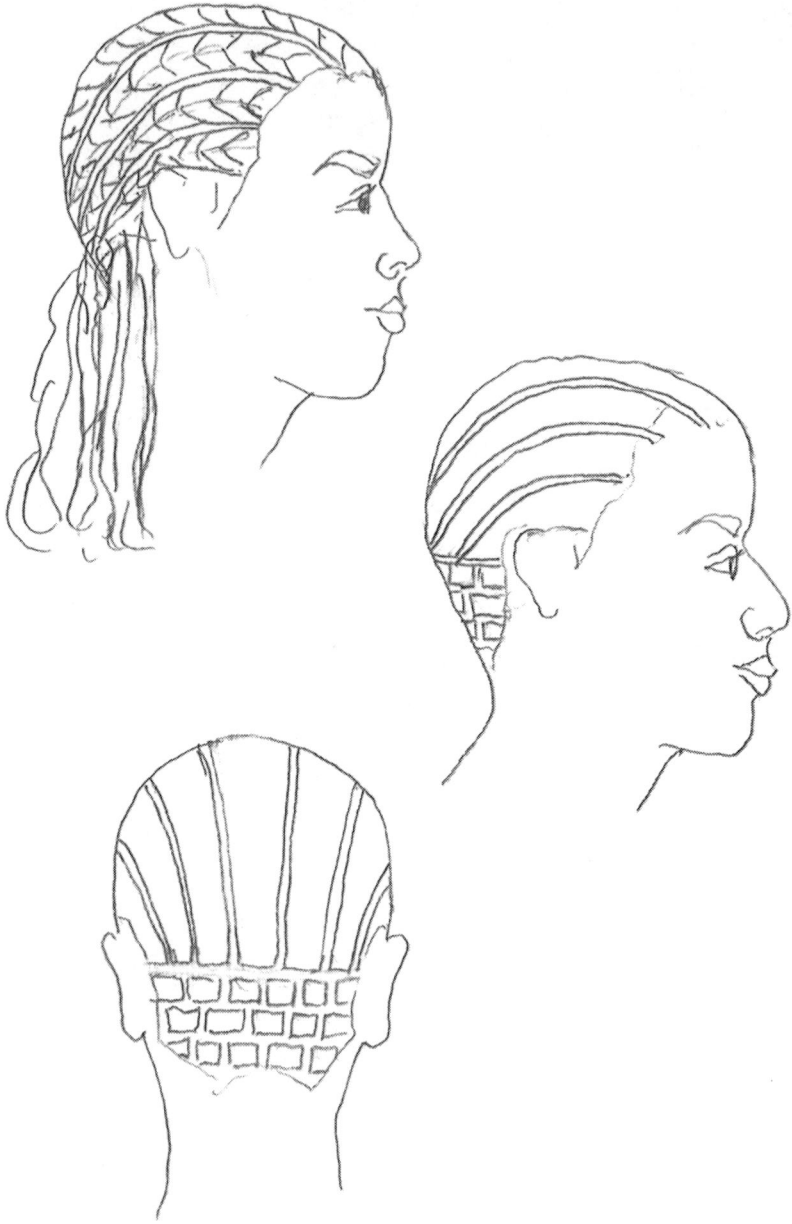

The hairstyle on the left is similar to an Ethiopian hairstyle that I saw on an educational channel once. The hairstyle here has two sections. The upper section is French braided. The lower back section consists of three rows of plaits. In the Ethiopian version, the hair was French braided front to back, without the three rows of plaits.

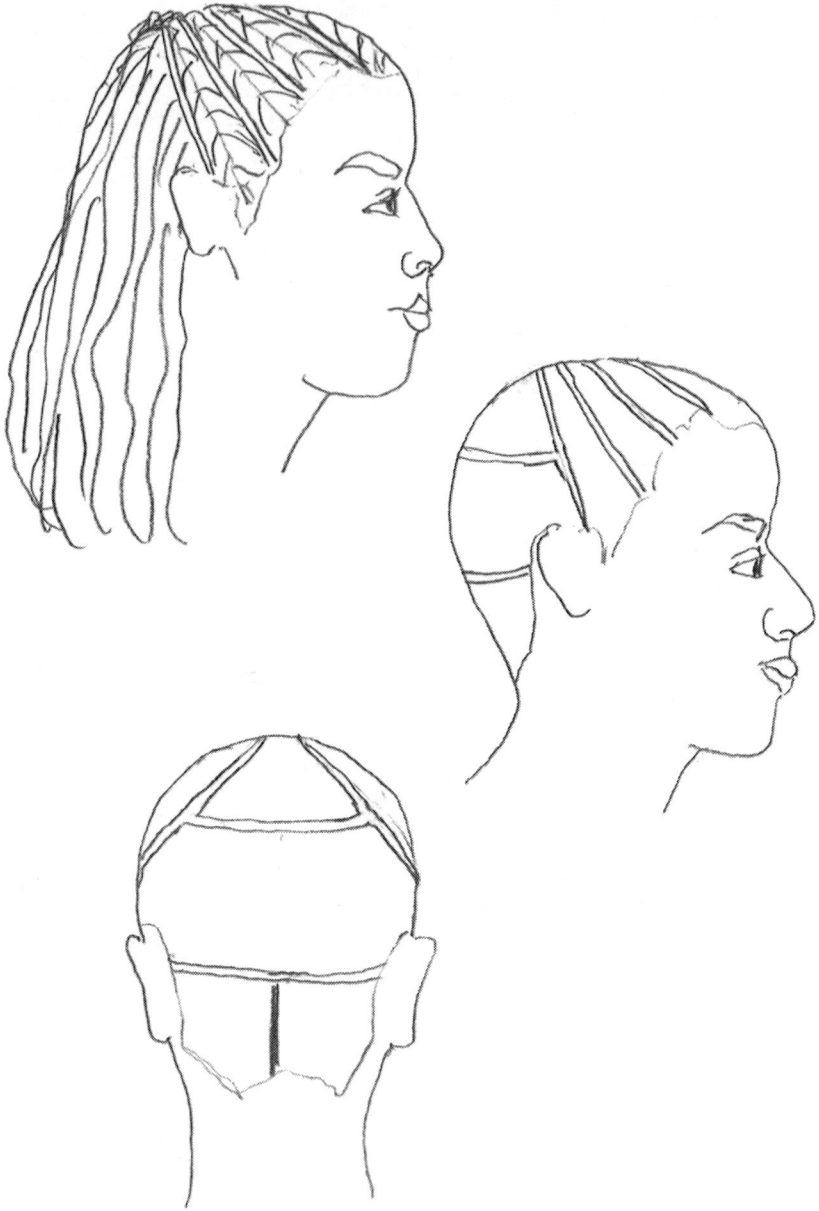

The hairstyle on the left has four sections. The front section is French braided. The back three sections in the finished style may be either in braids, plaits, or remain loose.

8
Your Personal Hair-care Diary

Keeping records is a tool to help monitor growth and development in any area of study. Use the following pages to sketch your own hairstyles, keep a record of your progress from month to month, and make notes on what works for you and what doesn't work for you.

Once you find the perfect combination of ingredients, you'll be glad that you kept note of such things as where a product was purchased, the date the product was purchased, cost, and anything else that will help you in getting to know your hair.

Year One Calendar

January						20_____
S	M	T	W	T	F	S

February						20_____
S	M	T	W	T	F	S

March						20_____
S	M	T	W	T	F	S

April						20_____
S	M	T	W	T	F	S

May						20_____
S	M	T	W	T	F	S

June						20_____
S	M	T	W	T	F	S

July						20_____
S	M	T	W	T	F	S

August						20_____
S	M	T	W	T	F	S

September						20_____
S	M	T	W	T	F	S

October						20_____
S	M	T	W	T	F	S

November						20_____
S	M	T	W	T	F	S

December						20_____
S	M	T	W	T	F	S

Your Color-Coded Legend:

trim split ends

wash

deep condition

rebraid

Year One Milestone Notes

Date: _____

Activity: _____

Comments: _____

_____

_____

Date: _____

Activity: _____

Comments: _____

_____

_____

_____

Date: _____

Activity: _____

Comments: _____

_____

_____

_____

Year Two Calendar

January	20_____

S	M	T	W	T	F	S

February	20_____

S	M	T	W	T	F	S

March	20_____

S	M	T	W	T	F	S

April	20_____

S	M	T	W	T	F	S

May	20_____

S	M	T	W	T	F	S

June	20_____

S	M	T	W	T	F	S

July	20_____

S	M	T	W	T	F	S

August	20_____

S	M	T	W	T	F	S

September	20_____

S	M	T	W	T	F	S

October	20_____

S	M	T	W	T	F	S

November	20_____

S	M	T	W	T	F	S

December	20_____

S	M	T	W	T	F	S

Your Color-Coded Legend:

- trim split ends
- wash
- deep condition
- rebraid

Year Two Milestone Notes

Date: _____

Activity: _____

Comments: _____

_____

_____

_____

Date: _____

Activity: _____

Comments: _____

_____

_____

_____

Date: _____

Activity: _____

Comments: _____

_____

_____

_____

Year Three Calendar

January					20___
S	M	T	W	T	F	S

February					20___
S	M	T	W	T	F	S

March					20___
S	M	T	W	T	F	S

April					20___
S	M	T	W	T	F	S

May					20___
S	M	T	W	T	F	S

June					20___
S	M	T	W	T	F	S

July					20___
S	M	T	W	T	F	S

August					20___
S	M	T	W	T	F	S

September					20___
S	M	T	W	T	F	S

October					20___
S	M	T	W	T	F	S

November					20___
S	M	T	W	T	F	S

December					20___
S	M	T	W	T	F	S

Your Color-Coded Legend:

	trim split ends
	wash
	deep condition
	rebraid
	_____
	_____
	_____
	_____

Year Three Milestone Notes

Date: _____

Activity: _____

Comments: _____

_____

_____

_____

Date: _____

Activity: _____

Comments: _____

_____

_____

_____

Date: _____

Activity: _____

Comments: _____

_____

_____

_____

Year Four Calendar

January	20____
February	20____
March	20____

S	M	T	W	T	F	S

April	20____
May	20____
June	20____

July	20____
August	20____
September	20____

October	20____
November	20____
December	20____

Your Color-Coded Legend:

	trim split ends
	wash
	deep condition
	rebraid

Year Four Milestone Notes

Date: _____

Activity: _____

Comments: _____

_____

_____

_____

Date: _____

Activity: _____

Comments: _____

_____

_____

_____

Date: _____

Activity: _____

Comments: _____

_____

_____

_____

Your Hairstyles and Notes

Your Hairstyles and Notes

Your Hairstyles and Notes

Your Hairstyles and Notes

Your Hairstyles and Notes

Your Hairstyles and Notes

Your Hairstyles and Notes

Your Hairstyles and Notes

Your Hairstyles and Notes

Your Hairstyles and Notes

Glossary

Following are definitions for words as used in this book that are unique to this book.

–A–

African braiding: The process of plaiting the hair down to the scalp by using the underhand method of plaiting the hair, and including hair from the side/beneath of a slice.

–B–

Base: At the scalp.

Bottom of the slice: Where African braiding or French braiding ends and plaiting begins.

Bound end(s): Refers to how fiber is packaged. Synthetic fiber is bound at the top and bottom; the top is the bound end, and the bottom is the free end. Human fiber is usually bound only at the top, the free end being loose.

Braid(s), braided, braiding, braiding process: Used interchangeably in this book. Depending on the context of the sentence, it can refer to African braids, French braids, plaits, or extensions, as opposed to simply braids.

Buildup: A combination of dust, natural scalp oil, grease, sweat, dead skin cells, lint, etc., which can combine to weaken and damage hair. Buildup also can cause matting. Buildup occurs most heavily near the base.

–C–

Clippers: Electric scissors used for cutting the hair; also known as shears.

Cornrows: This term and the term braids are used interchangeably as they both generally refer to the same hairstyling method.

CURB: Correctly Using Rubber Bands. This is the system invented by my sister to reduce hair breakage and hair loss that can be attributed to incorrectly using rubber bands on the hair.

Curly perm: One of two types of chemical treatments that African-Americans might use on their hair. The term refers to hair that has been permanently curled a specific diameter. This is achieved by using a chemical solution, so that the hair will not revert to its original state. The diameter of the curl is based on the diameter of the cold curler used on the hair during the chemical process. The other type of chemical treatment is known as a perm.

Cut bulk: Fiber that has been cut to a desired length in preparation for braiding.

–E–

Extensions: Fiber that has been interwoven into real hair.

–F–

Fiber: All false hair, whether synthetic or human.

Free end(s): The bottom of the length of fiber or hair.

French braid: The process of plaiting the hair down to the scalp by using the overhand method of plaiting the hair and including hair from the sides of a slice.

–H–

Hair type: In most cultural groups, different hair types can be found. For example, hair types among African-Americans vary from, and may be a combination of, hair that is (as defined in this book): body straight, which refers to hair that has a slight curl near the scalp, but other than that curl, the hair grows straight; bone straight, which refers to hair that has no body whatsoever, or potential for a natural curl; loose curls, which refers to hair in which the diameter of the curls is one-fourth inch or larger; tight curls, which refers to hair in which the diameter of the curls is less than three-sixteenths of an inch, and the individual hairs form a tight coil that sometimes reverses into a half curl along the length of the hair; and/or, loose or tight waves, which refers to hair that does not actually curl, but appears to alternately half-curl in one direction and then the opposite direction (in the shape of an "S") with the free ends of the hair (usually) appearing to actually curl. Wavy hair may half-curl either side to side, where the hairs lie flat on the scalp; or, the hair may appear to half-curl up and down, where the hairs stand up and away from the scalp.

–*K*–

Kinky: This word generally refers to anything abnormal, weird, bizarre, deviant in behavior, etc. note: I believe that using this word to describe an African-American hair type may subliminally enforce negative stereotypes, low self-esteem, and negative self-image.

–*L*–

Locs, locks: This is a hairstyle that originated with Rastafarians. It has been refined by African-Americans. The original hairstyle was called dreadlocks (please see the note on Kinky). The history of how the dreadlock hairstyle came to be is interesting, as is the Ras Tafari name, but it will not be covered in this book. In the Rastafarian version, individual hairs are allowed to tangle and grow in long, uncontrolled strands, resulting in a hairstyle where some strands are thicker than other strands. In the African-American version of this hairstyle, hair is grown out in a controlled fashion. The hair, as in the Rastafarian version, is deliberately allowed to tangle so that it "locks" up to the point that it cannot be easily untangled, and combed. In the African-American version, the hair is deliberately parted into small sections similar to small plaits, and then it is deliberately rolled and twisted between the fingers to help the hair begin to lock. An even more refined version of locs, which was developed by Dr. JoAnne Cornwell, is called "Sisterlocks."

–*M*–

Main part: Braided styles may be slanted, horizontal, or perpendicular to the wearers' shoulders. Main sections are subdivided during the braiding process to insure that the braids of the section being braided either slant, or are straight up and down—for example, to achieve the desired effect of the chosen style. This is usually accomplished by the strategic placement of one or more main parts.

Main sections: All braided styles can be sectioned off for volume (layers) or more control during the braiding process. These sections are then plaited or bobby-pinned out of the way while the braider works on one section at a time.

Matting: When braids have been in for some time without rebraiding, especially plaits, they may begin to look like a hairstyle called locs (can also be spelled as locks) that is worn by some Rastafarians. The appearance is that the hairs of the braid or plait seem to grow as one piece, or strand, of hair.

–N–

Nappy hair: Uncombed, or severely tangled hair.

–O–

Overhand plaiting: A method of styling the hair whereby a lock of hair is separated into three strands. Two adjacent strands are then twisted over each other. The third strand is then similarly twisted with the center strand. The process is then repeated. This method of plaiting the hair is the basis of all French braided hairstyles.

–P–

Perm, permanent, permed: One of two types of chemical treatments that African-Americans might use on their hair. The hair is permanently straightened (permed) by using a chemical solution so that it will not revert to its original state. The other type of chemical treatment is known as a curly perm.

Plait: A method of styling the hair whereby a lock of hair is separated into three strands. Two adjacent strands are then either twisted over or under each other. The third strand is then similarly twisted with the center strand. The process is then repeated. Twisting the strands over each other is known as overhand plaiting. Twisting the strands under each other is known as underhand plaiting.

Press, pressing: The hair is temporarily straightened using a special metal comb, heat, and a pressing creme or hair grease.

-R-

Retouch, retouching: When a perm is applied to the hair, its effects are permanent only on the hair on which the perm is applied. To keep the hair consistent in hair type, and to avoid breakage, a new perm is applied, based on the manufacturer's suggestions, to any hair that has grown out since the initial/last perm. This is called retouching the hair.

-S-

Scrunchies: Fabric-covered elastic.

Seam ripper: This is a sewing instrument used by seamstresses/tailors to remove (rip) stitches from fabric.

Slice: Refers to the hair to be braided, as in the hair between two parallel parts, or the hair between the hairline and a part parallel to it.

Strand(s): In braiding, the strip is usually divided into three parts; each part is considered one strand.

Strip: The initial lock of hairs that are separated from the slice in preparation for braiding. When plaiting the hair, the strip and the slice are usually one and the same.

-T-

Tightly curled hair: The hair type that is frequently, and incorrectly, referred to as kinky hair. This hair type has a tight, coil-type structure that sometimes reverses into a half curl along the individual hairs.

Too tight: Hair that has been braided too close to the scalp. Over time, hair that has been repeatedly braided too tightly may cause hair loss in the area.

Trim: To cut one-fourth inch to one-half inch from the ends of your hair.

-U-

Underhand plaiting: A method of styling the hair whereby a lock of hair is separated into three strands. Two adjacent strands are then twisted under each other. The third strand is then similarly twisted with the center strand. The process is then repeated. This method of plaiting the hair is the basis of all African braided hairstyles.

Wash: To shampoo and condition the hair.
Wean: To slowly stop using hair grease on the scalp.

Further Reading and Study

The following have not been used as references for this book; I've listed them for your information. I may, or may not, agree with some points of view contained within their pages or on their Web sites; however, I do believe that they all contain information that might help you to become a better braider, give you some insight into the African-American culture, or help you to grow as a Christian.

Since this is not a reference section in the traditional sense of the word, I've listed the name of the book first, then the author. On the next line you will find the ISBN (International Standard Book Number) for the book, which is used by booksellers and libraries to locate books they may wish to order. Anything written after the ISBN line is a tidbit from me about something that may have stood out to me about the book.

Books

1. *African Art* by Frank Willett
   ISBN-13: 9780500202678
2. *African Art in Cultural Perspective: An Introduction* by William Bascom
   ISBN-13: 9780393093759
3. *Ananse: The Web of Life in Africa* by John Biggers
   ISBN-13: 9781574412208

4. *Beautiful Black Hair: Real Solutions to Real Problems* by Shamboosie
   ISBN-13: 9780970222466
5. *Black Hair: Art, Style, and Culture* by Ima Ebong
   ISBN-13: 9780789306241
6. *The Black Woman's Guide to Beautiful Hair: A Positive Approach to Managing Any Hair and Style* by Lisa Akbari
   ISBN-13: 9781570719059
   A glance at Akbari's table of contents reveals an interesting chapter titled "Your Mind."
7. *Cornrows* by Camille Yarbrough
   ISBN-13: 9780698207097
   Yarbrough's book was written for children, but adults may find it interesting, too.
8. *Hair Matters: Beauty, Power, and Black Women's Consciousness* by Dr. Ingrid Banks
   ISBN-13: 9780814713372
9. *Hair Raising: Beauty, Culture, and African American Women* by Noliwe M. Rooks
   ISBN-13: 9780813523125
10. *Hair Story: Untangling the Roots of Black Hair in America* by Ayana D. Byrd, and Lori L. Tharps
    ISBN-13: 9780312283223
11. *Hairtalk: Stylish Braids from African Roots* by Duyan James
    ISBN-13: 9781402742354
12. *nappy: Growing Up Black and Female in America* by aliona l. gibson
    ISBN-13: 9780863163296
    This book has a wonderful chapter on the author's relationship with her hair and her self-image.
13. *Race Matters* by Dr. Cornel West
    ISBN-13: 9780679749868

14. *Vision of Beauty: The Story of Sarah Breedlove Walker* by Kathryn Lasky
    ISBN-13: 9780763602536
    This is a picture book for young children. It is the story of Madam C. J. Walker. The cover alone will make you want to read this book.
15. *When Reality Shines* by Susan Majette
    ISBN-13: 9780979875625 (revised edition)
    Written by the cousin of one of my cousins, this is an interesting book about surviving systemic lupus erythematosus, which includes how the author dealt with hair loss due to that disease. Majette's ending will surprise you.

Web Sites not Previously Noted

1. 700 Club, The
   http://www.cbn.org/
2. Braids by Breslin
   http://www.braidsbybreslin.com/
   I discovered this site after I constructed my Web site (www.dianakmitchell.com) for this book. Although she is a hair braider, Breslin does lace-front wigs too, and it is important to note why.
3. Center for Cultural Design
   http://www.ccd.rpi.edu/Eglash/csdt/african/CORNROW_CURVES/culture/african.origins.htm
   This site has a wonderful history of braiding, and has some good information about cornrow curves.
4. Christin Broadcasting Network
   http://www.ob.org/orphanspromise/index.asp
   This is the 700 Club's Web site for Operation Blessing's Orphan's Promise project. Donations benefit orphans around the world.
5. Travel the Road
   http://www.traveltheroad.com/
   This is a very engaging, and inspiring ministry site. It offers DVDs of the travels of two missionaries spreading the Gospel, Tim Scott, and Will Decker. They recently completed "Travel the Road: Season Three... Africa."

6. Trinity Broadcasting Network
   http://www.tbn.org
   This is a Christian network that offers a variety of Christian programming.
7. U.S. Census Bureau, The
   http://www.census.gov/
   Search "Table MS-3. Interracial Married Couples: 1980 to 2002." You might also perform searches on interracial and African-American.

Index

Note: Page entries followed by an "f" indicate that the reference is to a figure

French braiding, 24f
 African braiding versus, 26
 methods for extending. See French hair braid extension methods
 methods of, 25
 plaiting and. See hair plaiting
French hair braid extension methods
 As you go, 30f, 31
 Under and go, 28f, 29

G

"Gallery of Hairstyles"
 hairstyle, anatomy of, 69, 71, 73, 79, 81, 83, 68f, 70f, 72f, 74f–78f, 80f, 82f
 purpose of, 65
 slice, strip, and strands, 66f, 67

H

hair
 braiding of. See hair braiding
 breakage, identifying, 45
 brushing, 50
 combing, methods of, 10, 11
 drying, methods of, 10–11
 exercises for healthy, 57
 growth, 4–5
 hairstylists, role of, 51
 healthy growth of, maintaining, 56
 human, 7
 plaiting. See hair plaiting
 synthetic, 7
 template of dairy for maintaining, 85–103
 tips to grow long, 6, 55–56
 types of, 7
 washing, methods of, 9–10, 56
Hair Braider's Secret Reference Manual, The (Mitchell), 62
hair braiding, 13
 African style of, 3. See also African braiding
 care for. See Braid care
 cut bulk preparations before, 15–16
 extensions, methods of using, 7–8

S

scarves, uses of, 46
seam ripper
      method for using, 45
      utility of, 44, 45
shadowing technique, 59–60
synthetic hair. See fiber

T

"Table MS-3. Interracial Married Couples: 1980 to 2002," (U.S.
      Census Bureau), 1–2
Tyson, Cicely, 3–4

U

Under and around method, 18f, 19
Under and go method
      for African braiding, 20f, 21
      for French braiding method, 28f, 29
Underplait extension-plaiting, 36f, 37

W

Warren, Pastor Rick, 62
Woodson, Julie, 4

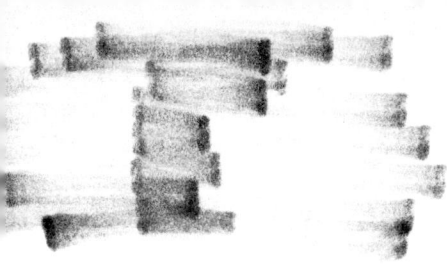

DATE DUE

780595 523504